Computer
Analysis of
Neuronal Structures

Computers in Biology and Medicine

Series Editor: George P. Moore
University of Southern California, Los Angeles

COMPUTER ANALYSIS OF NEURONAL STRUCTURES
Edited by Robert D. Lindsay

In preparation:

INFORMATION TECHNOLOGY IN HEALTH SCIENCE EDUCATION
Edited by Edward C. Deland

COMPUTER-ASSISTED EYE EXAMINATION
Edited by Elwin Marg

A Continuation Order Plan is available for this series. A continuation order will bring delivery of each new volume immediately upon publication. Volumes are billed only upon actual shipment. For further information please contact the publisher.

Computer
Analysis of
Neuronal Structures

Edited by
Robert D. Lindsay
University of California, Los Angeles

Plenum Press · New York and London

1977

Library of Congress Cataloging in Publication Data

Main entry under title:

Computer analysis of neuronal structures.
  (Computers in biology and medicine)
  Includes bibliographies and index.
  1. Neuroanatomy–Data Processing. 2. Neurons. I. Lindsay, Robert D. II. Series:
Computers in biology and medicine (New York, 1977-   )
QL931.C66   591.4'8   76-50605
ISBN 0-306-30964-5

© 1977 Plenum Press, New York
A Division of Plenum Publishing Corporation
227 West 17th Street, New York, N.Y. 10011

Dedicated to the memory of

Donald Arthur Sholl

Contributors

P. J. R. Boyle, Department of Anatomy, University of Colorado Medical Center, Denver, Colorado 80220

Christopher Brown, Department of Computer Science, University of Rochester, Rochester, New York 14627

M. Chujo, Department of Physiology and Biophysics, New York University Medical Center, 550 First Avenue, New York, New York 10016

Paul D. Coleman, Department of Anatomy, University of Rochester Medical Center, Rochester, New York 14642

R. F. Dunn, Department of Surgery, UCLA School of Medicine, Los Angeles, California 90024; and Department of Otolaryngology, University of Pittsburgh School of Medicine, Pittsburgh, Pennsylvania 15213

Catherine F. Garvey, Department of Anatomy and Division of Biomathematics, University of Rochester Medical Center, Rochester, New York 14642

Sheryl Glasser, Department of Biology, University of California San Diego, La Jolla, California 92093

E. Harth, Physics Department, Syracuse University, Syracuse, New York 13210

D. E. Hillman, Department of Physiology and Biophysics, New York University Medical Center, 550 First Avenue, New York, New York 10016

W. E. Kumley, Department of Surgery, UCLA School of Medicine, Los Angeles, California 90024; and Department of Otolaryngology, University of Pittsburgh School of Medicine, Pittsburgh, Pennsylvania

Robert D. Lindsay, Brain Research Institute and Department of Anatomy, University of California School of Medicine, Los Angeles, California 90024

R. Llinás, Department of Physiology and Biophysics, New York University Medical Center, 550 First Avenue, New York, New York 10016

John Miller, Department of Biology, University of California San Diego, La Jolla, California 92093

D. P. O'Leary, Department of Surgery, UCLA School of Medicine, Los Angeles, California 90024

A. Paldino, Department of Neuroscience, Rose Fitzgerald Kennedy Center for Research in Mental Retardation and Human Development, Albert Einstein College of Medicine, Bronx, New York 10461

Allen Selverston, Department of Biology, University of California San Diego, La Jolla, California 92093

William Simon, Division of Biomathematics, University of Rochester Medical Center, Rochester, New York 14642

D. G. Whitlock, Department of Anatomy, University of Colorado Medical Center, Denver, Colorado 80220

N. G. Xuong, Department of Biology, University of California San Diego, La Jolla, California 92093

John H. Young, Division of Biomathematics, University of Rochester Medical Center, Rochester, New York 14642

Foreword

It seems particularly appropriate that this pioneering collection of papers should be dedicated to Donald Sholl since those of us who count, measure, and reconstruct elements of the neural ensemble are all very much in his debt. Sholl was certainly not the first to attempt quantification of certain aspects of brain structure. No computers were available to him for the kind of answers he sought, and some of his answers — or rather his interpretations — may not stand the test of time. But we remember him because of the questions he asked and for the reasons he asked them.

At a time when the entire family of Golgi techniques was in almost total eclipse, he had the judgment to rely on them. And in a period when the canonical neuron was a perfect sphere (the enormous dendritic superstructure being almost forgotten), he was one of a very few who looked to dendrite extension and pattern as a prime clue to the overall problem of neuronal connectivity.

As we have said, Sholl was not the first to attempt to introduce some degree of quantification into descriptions of the nervous system. Even before the turn of the century, Donaldson, in his book *The Growth of the Brain* (University of Chicago Press, Chicago, 1895), developed figures for total cortical area and volume, and for the presumed numbers of neurons making up the mass of the cortical mantle. Both problems were formidable ones at the time and, even today, present challenging technical difficulties. These are evidenced by the order-of-magnitude differences which can be found in estimates by workers such as von Economo and Koskinas, Agduhr, Rowland and Mettler, and Shariff. Various techniques were used by these investigators, including direct counting from the microscope and counts made from photomicrographs and from projected images. In all of these methods, major problems revolved about the proper treatment of the depth factor. Sections thin enough to be handled as two-dimensional surfaces clearly cut through cells and nuclei in massive if indeterminate numbers. Sections thick enough to provide reasonable numbers of intact somata necessitated study under conditions of continual focusing through depth, with the added uncertainty of how to select, or reject, nuclei cut through at both tissue interfaces. While there is probably no completely satisfactory solution to this problem, Sholl called attention to a correction factor proposed by Abercrombie in 1946 which at least took this factor into account. From this he developed, on a layer-by-layer basis, values for the density of neuronal packing, a parameter which has assumed increasing importance as a possible clue to "quality" of the cortical cell matrix.

Probably the two most significant ideas which are associated with Sholl are the quantitative description of the dendritic tree and the connective zone of the neuron. Both of these concepts are elaborations of earlier ones proposed by Bok (*Histonomy of the Cerebral Cortex*, Elsevier, Amsterdam, 1959). Sholl demonstrated that the successive branching patterns of each dendrite tree could be described graphically if the dendrite domain was superimposed on a set of concentric spheres centering, in most cases, on the soma. The pattern of dendrite—sphere interactions plotted against distance from the perikaryon suggested an exponential function of the general form $y = ae^{-kx}$, where x represented distance from the perikaryon. The eventual interest of such a relationship might then reside in its ability to describe changes in density of the dendritic domain from inside out and, as a result, the probability of such a neuron being affected by impulses traveling along fibers in its vicinity. He assumed that each dendritic branch of the domain (and of soma) was surrounded by a sleeve of space — the connective zone — approximately 0.5 μm wide. Any axon found in this space would be considered a potential synaptic contact.

> ... Between any consecutive pair of the spherical shells that were previously mentioned, there will be a volume of cortex, say V, that will contain a connective zone of volume T. The ration [sic] T/V can be computed from the data and will be called the regional connective field density. For the stellate cells and for the basal dendrites of the pyramids, the connective field density decays exponentially with the distance from the perikaryon except in the immediate neighborhood of the perikaryon, where the volume of the connective zone is enormously increased by the presence of the perikaryon. The order of this decay can be illustrated by the connective field density of a stellate cell, which is given by $k \cdot exp(-0.035x)$, x being the distance from the perikaryon.
>
> These results show that it is not only possible to classify the neurons in accordance with a qualitative description of their modes of connectivity, but it is possible to give a quantitative indication of the extent to which a single neuron may be influenced by impulses travelling in its neighborhood (Sholl, D., *The Organization of the Cerebral Cortex*, Methuen, London, 1956, pp. 55–57).

From this type of analysis of cortical neurons and from somewhat similar considerations of the presynaptic elements impinging on these ensembles, he conceived that the overall scheme of connectional patterns among cortical elements could be described in statistical terms where the connections of individual neurons are of less concern than the general pattern of the neuronal aggregate.

Such a scheme appeared to represent a happy alternative to the specific connectional approach championed by Cajal and the classical Golgi anatomists. Certainly the formidable difficulties imposed by the latter could well have proven one of the factors contributing to the waning of the brilliant Golgi era of the late nineteenth century. However, the promised advantages of rigor and relative simplification implicit in Sholl's ideas did not go long unchallenged. The specificity of axodendritic connections on cortical cell spines was soon demonstrated by the electron microscope, in part by his University College colleague, George Gray, while the postulated random quality of connectional patterns became increasingly untenable following the resurgence of Golgi and reduced silver studies and the even greater rigor of microlesioning, radioautography, selective axonal transport techniques, etc. Sholl's concepts of connectional architectonics are clearly subject to considerable revamping, but his quantitative description of the dendritic envelope and his attempts at probabilistic modeling must remain significant scientific and historic milestones.

The contents of the present volume would certainly have proved of great interest to him. The mix of papers include theoretical discussion, presentations of the new computer-centered quantitative technology, and examples of the type of data to be derived from these methodologies. He would see that the Golgi methods remain prepotent in enabling presentation of the type of qualitative information upon which the new algorithms are built. At the same time it would be clear that the strengths of the methodology are such that tridimensional reconstructions of the electron microscopic image, as well as elaborate syntheses from instruments of even higher resolving power, lie just around the corner. And he would be fascinated by the quantal advances in analysis of field geometry and neuronal interconnections which have been made possible by modern computer speed and capacity . . . to say nothing of the virtuosity of solid-state circuitry and chip dynamics which bring all of these capabilities within range of the individual investigator in his laboratory. This is a book he would have enjoyed and read many times — if he had not written it!

We can recall our one brief contact with Don Sholl. We had finished nine months of work on single-unit activity with Moruzzi in Pisa and were on our way to see the Fessards in Paris and Brodal in Oslo. Following a week at Cambridge, we visited University College where J. Z. Young introduced us to Sholl as kindred spirits also wrestling with the brilliant but exasperating Golgi methods. We ended up spending two evenings with Sholl and his wife, testing the London cuisine along with the scientific waters. He was a quiet man, reserved, sometimes humorous, occasionally even sardonic. He talked a little about his earlier mathematical background and his recent essay into neurobiology. For his time, he was superbly equipped to do what he wished to do. And he laughed as we described our own attempts, while still working at the University of Tennessee at Memphis, to interest some of the faculty at Georgia Tech in developing mathematical relationships for us from a group of measurements we sent them on pre- and postsynaptic fields in inferior olive and cerebellum. "It's too soon," he told us. "It will take years for people to realize that there are other significantly measurable quantities in the central nervous system besides the total number of cells, nuclei, and nucleoli." We talked a little about organizing a symposium in the United States (where funds were more easily available) in a few years to cross fertilize with the few investigators then around who shared our belief in the significance of dendrites and their connectional patterns. Such a meeting might result in a written record (the examples of the brilliant Hixon and Laurentian symposia were fresh in our minds) which could in turn reintroduce others to the possibilities inherent in the dendritic domain.

But there was no meeting and we never saw him again. In less than three years he was dead.

Arnold and Madge Scheibel

Los Angeles

Preface

More and more quantitative description is being incorporated into neuro-anatomy as this science is being integrated with the other areas of neuroscience. This volume describes in detail the use of the laboratory computer to study the structure of the nervous system. This structure is immensely complex and its quantitative study will require a sophisticated approach.

The authors of this volume are pioneers in applying modern data-processing techniques to the study of neuronal structure. Several visualization methods have been utilized such as Golgi impregnation, dye injection, electron microscopy, autoradiography, and myelin staining. Although the approaches differ, the various authors have similar aims, and a common theme is evident throughout.

The book discusses the considerations in the development of automated data acquisition systems. The hardware and software of specific systems are described in detail. Included are the data acquisition and processing procedures. Several sections deal with the computer graphic presentation of structural data. Methods for quantitative analysis of neuronal structures are described using both statistical and analytical techniques. The book also outlines the general types of studies to be carried out using each system.

This volume is the result of conversations with George Moore, who is the series editor for *Computers in Biology and Medicine*. George and I have been close friends for some time and he has been enthusiastic about our techniques for quantitative neuronal reconstructions using computers. He suggested that we write a book on the quantitative methods of studying neuronal structure. From various publications and through personal contact at several society meetings, we were aware of other groups interested in a similar approach. Thus we were able to compile a comprehensive list of potential authors. Interest and enthusiasm for the book was high. We all felt that these new techniques should be presented from the point of view of the "working neuroscientist" rather than that of a clever engineering feat. We also agreed that the book should be dedicated to Donald Sholl.

I would like to extend my gratitude to the contributing authors for their excellent cooperation in putting this volume together and for the time taken away from other academic pursuits and their family activities.

My thanks to George Moore for launching me on this interesting literary adventure and being instrumental in bringing this endeavor smoothly to a conclusion. I would also like to cite the cooperation and support I received from Madge and Arnold Scheibel. It was greatly appreciated. I would like to especially mention Erich Harth, for it was he who originally encouraged me to undertake the quantitative structural analysis of the nervous system.

Every book requires a sacrifice of time and mental activity to bring an idea to the finished product. Usually it is the spouse and offspring who suffer the vented frustration or else endure isolation during the actual writing. Our case is no exception, but the burden was greatly reduced since I had the complete cooperation of my family. Barbara, my wife, has been an active participant in all phases of the preparation of this volume. The enthusiastic interest of my children, Robert, Bruce, and Brenda, in my neuronal "trees" has been a constant stimulus.

Robert D. Lindsay

Los Angeles

Contents

Chapter 10

Christopher Brown

Chapter 11

A. Paldino and E. Harth

Computer
Analysis of
Neuronal Structures

The Video Computer Microscope and A.R.G.O.S.

Robert D. Lindsay

1. Introduction

The structural study of neurons was begun about 1900 with the classical works of Santiago Ramon y Cajal, a Spanish neuroanatomist. Many contemporary neurohistologists still follow his method of drawing and describing the delicately impregnated neurons using the Golgi technique. Although this method has enormously advanced our understanding of the structure of central nervous systems, the method is subjective and, as a consequence, has led to many disputes among leading authorities in the field (Sholl, 1956).

One of the major factors in the disputes is the structural nature of the central nervous system and the histological techniques used to visualize the various components. The tissue of the central nervous system is packed with neurons having somata of various sizes and bifurcating processes which often extend for long distances. Threading through this network are afferent fibers from different distal sources which frequently branch. Such material would present special difficulties to the neurohistologist even if a good technique were found to make all the desired components of the nervous tissue visible. If a section is cut thick enough to include one neuron in its entirety, the result is such a bewildering maze of closely interwoven processes that structural analysis of the neuron is very difficult, if not impossible. Despite the difficulties, much has been learned about the structure of the central nervous system using a combination of histological techniques.

Another major problem that confronts the neurohistologist is that even a small portion of the central nervous system is composed of a large number of

Robert D. Lindsay · Brain Research Institute and Department of Anatomy, University of California School of Medicine, Los Angeles, California 90024.

heterogeneous elements. Recognizing that a purely descriptive method is inadequate, some neurohistologists are applying quantitative methods and statistical analysis to improve their description of structure. Progress in obtaining quantitative data has been slow because a great deal of effort and time are required to make even the crudest measurements on a small number of structures.

A very large amount of data is required to represent a structure as complicated as a neuron. The need for modern data-collecting and -processing methods is obvious. The central problem is how to convert microscopic images into a three-dimensional representation for computer analysis.

2. Histological Preparation

The silver impregnation technique introduced by the Italian neurohistologist Golgi in the 1870s is at present the most useful for the quantitative structural study of neurons in mammalian brain tissue. When tissue is prepared using this technique, a select few neurons are opaquely impregnated in their entirety against a pale yellow background. The mechanism of the technique is unknown and the results are unpredictable. It has been widely used for the qualitative study of neurons for many years and has been invaluable.

Since the time of Golgi, many have made modifications in his dichromate-silver technique. The most important modification of the technique was made by Golgi himself: the addition of osmic acid to the dichromate solution. Axons, their collaterals, and dendrites are impregnated with a delicacy that has not been surpassed with any of the other modifications (Ramon-Moliner, 1957). The addition of osmic acid to the chromating solution also reduces the chromating period. Hence this modification is known as the *rapid Golgi technique*. Although the rapid Golgi technique has a high reliability of impregnating axons and their collaterals, the method frequently gives patchy results with regard to the distribution of somata. The distribution of impregnation is dependent not only on the histological procedure but also on the kind of animal, type of tissue, and geometric blocking of the tissue. Even when all these factors are taken into account, the resulting distribution can be unpredictable.

The following procedure has been successfully used to prepare histological preparations for quantitative structural studies of neurons: Brains were prepared for examination by perfusion with normal saline and Lillie's neutral buffered formalin (McManus and Mowry, 1960). The brain tissue was additionally fixed in formalin for 2 days. Each brain was then divided into blocks having a thickness of less than 4 mm. The blocks of tissue were placed in the rapid Golgi chromating solution for 3 days. The blocks of tissue were then placed in a

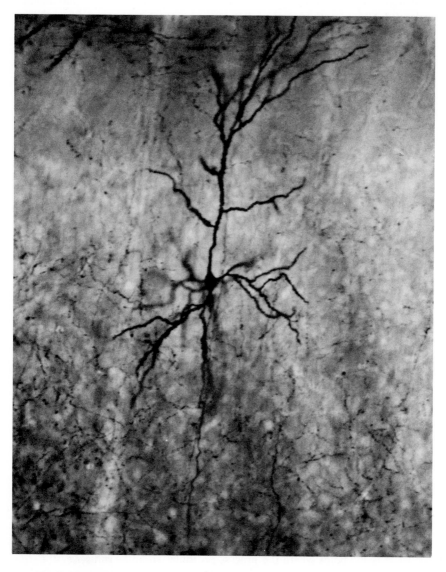

Fig. 1. Photomicrograph of a neuron impregnated using the rapid Golgi technique.

silvering solution for 24 hr. The blocks of tissue were dehydrated and embedded in Parlodion (Davenport, 1960). The blocks were serially sliced on a sliding microtome at a thickness of 100–200 μm, and the tissue slices were mounted on slides using Permount and coverglasses.

Serial slices carefully prepared by this method have been used to trace individual fibers from one slice to the next. This technique makes possible the complete reconstruction of the dendritic domain and as much of the axonal domain as is desired (Lindsay, 1971). Figure 1 is a photomicrograph of a neuron impregnated using the rapid Golgi technique.

3. Structural Data Model

In order for the quantitative approach to reach its full potential in the study of neuronal morphology, the experimental measurements must be comprehensive. Since most mammalian neurons have a complex structure, associating a few numbers with a neuron does not give a good representation of the structure. What is needed is a data model that approximates the complex structure up to a certain degree of resolution. This method has been referred to as *neuronal reconstruction.*

As already stated, neurons consist of a few fibrous processes which protrude from a soma. The processes bifurcate into an arbor in a manner similar to that of the branches of trees. One data model used to represent the bifurcating fibrous structure of dendrites and axons is the "stick" or "wire" model (Harth and Lindsay, 1968; Lindsay, 1971; Wann *et al.*, 1973). The three-dimensional coordinates in space are given for each each inflection, branch, and end point. A code associated with the coordinates of the point and the sequential order of the points determine the connectivity of the points and hence the sticklike structure.

The data model consists of a sequence of points. Each point consists of four numbers of which three are the three-dimensional coordinates in space and the fourth is a code that classifies the point. Four major types of points are necessary to represent a treelike structure: a beginning point or the *root* of the tree, branching points or the *nodes*, and end points or *termini*. Since fibers do not project in a straight line, inflection points are used to indicate the curvature. The order of the points is crucial to the representation. The first point in the sequence is the point where the process protrudes from the soma, i.e., the root, followed by inflection points to a node. The sequence of points continues along one branch to other nodes until a terminus is encountered. At this point, the sequence continues from the previous node. The sequence of points continues in the same manner until the entire structure is represented. Figure 2 is an example of the sequence of points. Note that it is arbitrary which branch one proceeds along and the sequence is not unique in that several sequences can represent the same structure.

This scheme for recording structural data of neuronal processes has the advantage of requiring a minimal amount of information, or in our case computer memory, for the desired structure. Further, subsequent data processing is easily performed and three-dimensional information presents no special problems to this scheme.

This stick model can be expanded to include varying fiber diameters by adding a fifth number to the point. Also, special points may be added to represent spines and nodules, thus increasing the data content of the model.

The number of *points* needed to represent the structure of a small pyramidal cell is between 500 and 800. Thus 2000–3200 *numbers* are required to represent the structure of a single neuron. If one wished to extract even a simple specific parameter from these data, the arithmetic manipulation of such a mass of numbers would represent an astronomical task, not to mention the measurements involved. Clearly some sort of automated system is needed for the collection and processing of the structural data of neurons.

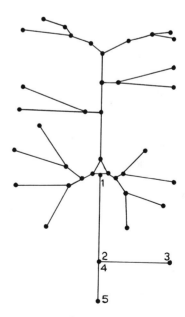

Fig. 2. Simplified stick figure representing the measured data. Each dot indicates a three-dimensional coordinate point. A code associated with each point is used to signify inflection, branch, or end point. The points are numbered to indicate the sequence in which they would be measured.

4. *System Design Considerations*

A number of general requirements should be considered in the development of a system for the acquisition of neuronal structural data. First, the three-dimensional representation of the entire neuron should be possible, even though the structure is contained in several serial tissue sections. Second, the structural information should be passed from the histological image to the computer with a minimum of effort and without hand recording of the data. Third, the structural data should be in a form such that they can be used for a variety of analysis procedures. Fourth, the major hardware components for such a system should be commercially available and a minimum of special components should be necessary. Finally the expenses of the system should be minimized to make it available to a number of investigators.

One of the early considerations in the development of a data-acquisition system for neuronal structure is the choice of an automatic or a semiautomatic system. An automatic system is defined as a system that acquires and stores the structural data of a neuron from histological preparations without intervention of an operator. Two general schemes for automatic systems have been explored. The first scheme utilizes a *beam-scanning* technique similar to television (Ledley, 1964; Reddy *et al.*, 1973). The entire visual image is converted into a series of discrete intensity levels and stored in computer memory. These systems have the disadvantage of requiring very large and expensive computer systems to store and process the image data. Also, the collected data are not in a convenient form for neuronal structural analysis. Special pattern-recognition algorithms are necessary for neuronal reconstruction. But perhaps the largest problem is the difficulty in treating three-dimensional objects.

The second general scheme for an automatic system utilizes the principle of *autotracking* (Garvey *et al.*, 1973). Since the image of a Golgi-impregnated neuron is a continuous pattern, a complete tracking over the entire structure is possible. This scheme has the advantage of being able to track a neuronal fiber in three dimensions. The tracking control and data acquisition can utilize the less expensive laboratory-size computer. The disadvantage of this scheme has been the very special equipment required. The development of such equipment can be expensive and time consuming. Recently, hardware components have become commerically available that could be used to assemble an automatic system using the autotracking scheme.

Most investigators interested in applying modern data-collecting techniques to the study of neuronal structure have selected the semiautomatic scheme. The rationale for such systems is to divide the tasks between the operator and computer, permitting both to do what they do best. Thus the operator performs the pattern recognition portion and indicates where measurements are to be made, while the manipulation, computation, and storage of the data are accomplished by the computer. These systems have the advantage of being assembled from commercially available components. They are relatively inexpensive. The data are in a form easily analyzed for structure. Also, three-dimensional reconstruction presents no special problem. The disadvantage is the amount of time necessary to record the structure of a single neuron, thus limiting the scope of a study.

5. Video Computer Microscope

An automated data-acquisition system for the quantitative reconstruction of Golgi-impregnated neurons was developed by the author at UCLA. The hardware portion of this system is referred to as the *video computer microscope* (VCM). The system is used to collect data in the form of a stick model to represent the branching structure of neuronal processes. Specifically, the system was designed to extract a sequence of spatial points from histological preparations to represent structure.

The acquisition of structural data from microscopic structures such as neurons requires a high-magnification optical device. This system uses a Leitz ortholux II binocular research microscope equipped with a phototube and achromatic dry plano objectives. A Shibaden CCTV camera is mounted above the microscope and is optically coupled to the phototube. The video signal from the CCTV camera is sent to a 17-inch CCTV monitor (see Fig. 3).

Measurement of the x and y coordinates of a point on the screen of the CCTV monitor is accomplished using a GRAF/PEN. This device is comprised of three components: an L-frame sensor, a recording pen, and a controller. The L-frame is mounted on the CCTV monitor as seen in Fig. 4. The bars of the L-frame are strip microphones. When the pen is touched to the surface of the screen, an ultrasonic pulse is emitted and the time of flight is determined between the pen and nearest point to each microphone. Using the time of flight and the speed of sound, the distance is determined. The manufacturer claims a precision of 0.007 inch for these measurements. The two orthogonal distances are the x and y coordinates of a point on the screen. Binary registers for the x coordinate, the y coordinate, and a ready flag contained in the controller are connected to the digital inputs of the laboratory computer. The ready flag signals the computer that coordinates of a point have been determined and the data are ready to be read.

In order to determine the z coordinate, the optical condenser of the microscope is adjusted to give a narrow depth of field. Each point to be recorded is brought into best focus. The shaft of a potentiometer is coupled to the fine-focus control. The value of the potential across the potentiometer is directly proportional to the depth of the point in the slice of tissue. The potentiometer is electrically connected to an analog input of the computer. When the GRAF/PEN signals that a point has been measured, the computer samples the voltage at the analog input and thus determines the z coordinate of the point.

The fourth number to be associated with the x, y, z coordinates is the *point code*. The number of the code is entered by way of the CODE BOX, which consists of an array of 12 touch switches. Eight potentiometers connected to the analog inputs of the computer comprise the POT BOX. These potentiometers are used for the manual entry of parameters in the slice-matching procedure.

Two rows of lamp indicators connected to the digital outputs of the computer are mounted in the LIGHT BOX. These lamps are used to communicate to the operator which routines are currently being executed and which point code is to be entered next.

The central component of the video computer microscope is the Digital Equipment Corporation LAB-8/e laboratory computer. The configuration consists of a PDP-8/e processor, 16 K words of core memory, an extended

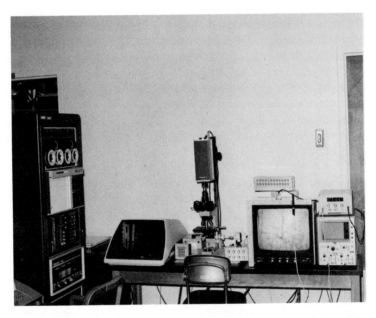

Fig. 3. Video computer microscope. The major components seen from left to right are the laboratory computer, the video terminal, the research microscope with a CCTV camera mounted above, the CCTV monitor with an L-frame sensor attached to the screen, and the oscilloscope with the GRAF/PEN controller above. The CODE BOX is to the left of the microscope and the POT BOX is to the right of the microscope. The LIGHT BOX is above the CCTV monitor.

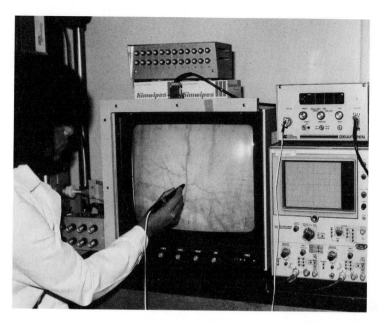

Fig. 4. CCTV monitor and the GRAF/PEN digitizing system.

arithmetic element, 8 channels of analog input, a programmable clock, a point-lot display control, three 12-bit digital inputs, three 12-bit digital outputs, a dual-drive DECtape unit, and a terminal interface. Either a video terminal or a standard teletype is used as the operator console for the computer. The video terminal provides a convenient console for the data-collection operation and the teletype is used for printed output of the analysis programs.

The point-plot display control is used for graphic display of data on an oscilloscope. Under program control, a bright spot can be momentarily produced at any point in a 1024 by 1024 array on the screen of the CRT. A series of these intensified dots can be programmed to produce graphic output. The graphic presentation is limited only by the extent of the programming the user desires to implement. The VCM uses the graphic display to present the operator with a visual representation of the collected data.

6. A.R.G.O.S.

The computer program used for the neuronal reconstruction is referred to as A.R.G.O.S. The acronym stands for *anatomical reconstruction graphics operating system*. The programming of a digital computer, referred to as the software, provides the creative construction of the automated system. Imagination and logical construction are especially important in the development of software involving man—machine interactions in real time. A.R.G.O.S. is such an interactive type of program. It aids the investigator with all functions required for neuronal reconstruction, except pattern recognition.

A.R.G.O.S. makes use of the *program interrupt facility* in order to share the computer processing between two tasks. The program interrupt facility allows certain external conditions to interrupt the execution of a computer program routine and initiate another routine. Every device able to request a program interrupt contains a special one-bit register called an *interrupt request flag*. When the interrupt facility is enabled and any device requests an interrupt, the computer automatically disables its interrupt facility and jumps to an interrupt service routine. The interrupt facility allows an ongoing routine, referred to as the *background program*, to continue until such time that a device signals that another routine, called a *foreground program*, is to be executed. Multiple-device interrupt programming requires a service routine that determines the source of an interrupt request. When the foreground routine is completed, the interrupt facility is reenabled and the computer executes a jump to resume the background program execution.

The background program for A.R.G.O.S. is a point-plot display of the measured structural data. This type of display requires the computer to continuously cycle through the display data in order to refresh the display on the screen. Two projected views of the structural data are presented on the display screen. In the middle of the left half of the screen is presented the *X-Y* plane projection of the structure. The right half of the screen is used to present the *Y-Z* plane projection of the structure. In both presentations, the *Y* axis is vertically oriented on the screen. Hence the relationship between the two projections is a 90° rotation about the vertical axis of the screen.

A.R.G.O.S. recognizes interrupts from three hardware devices, the console keyboard, the CODE BOX, and the GRAF/PEN. When a key on the console keyboard is pressed, the service routine is entered. The keyboard is recognized as the interrupting device, the key pressed is decoded, and the appropriate routine is entered. In the following discussion, the interactive data-acquisition procedure and the explanation of the foreground programs are described.

Before points are recorded for the reconstruction of the selected neuron, the output units of the GRAF/PEN must be related to the dimensions of the tissue. When "X" is pressed on the console, A.R.G.O.S. enters the *lateral magnification routine*. A glass micrometer slide is placed on the stage of the microscope. The console requests entry of the distance between two points seen on the monitor screen. The investigator responds by entering the number on the console and recording the two points using the GRAF/PEN. The procedure is carried out for all four objective lenses.

The potentiometer connected to the fine-focus control of the microscope yields a voltage proportional to the relative position of the control. The *Z-axis calibration routine* is entered by pressing "Z" on the console. The console requests the entry of the tissue slice number. After entry, the top surface is brought into best focus and then the RETURN key is pressed. Next the bottom surface is brought into best focus and the RETURN key is pressed.

During the data processing and analysis, the investigator will find it desirable to associate a number of descriptive parameters with the structural data of the selected neuron. The *associated cell data* routine is initiated by pressing "A" on the console keyboard. The console responds by requesting a keyboard or a GRAF/PEN entry. Some of the entries in the following example are specific to the cerebral cortex. For cells from other areas, other appropriate entries can be substituted for the cortical-specific entries. The first request is the assignment of a *cell identification number*. The source of brain tissue for the selected neuron is then identified by the *type* of brain, *area* location of the neuron, and *brain* and *tissue block* identification numbers. A *shrinkage factor* is entered to account for shrinkage of the tissue during fixation and subsequent processing. The *section orientation* and *slice thickness* are identified. An *experiment number* and a *group number* are included to classify and subclassify the selected neuron for analysis studies. A *procedure number* is used to identify the particular protocol used for the reconstruction.

The *cortical thickness* and *soma depth* at the location of the selected neuron are measured using the GRAF/PEN. The GRAF/PEN is also used to record three points for *orientation* of the neuron to the tissue section. The *cell type* and *number of processes* are included. The *diameter of the soma* is measured using the GRAF/PEN. The *slice of tissue* in which the soma is contained is identified. For pyramidal cells, the *apical dendrite* is identified. The selection of the *objective lens* for coordinate measurement is entered.

The *display option routine* is initiated by pressing "D" on the console keyboard. The console then requests the entry of the *display mode* and the *display magnification factor*. At the present time, the only mode of display implemented is the one previously described. The display array is consequently updated with the new magnification factor.

Once the lateral magnification, *Z* calibration, associated cell data entry, and display mode routines have been executed, the investigator is ready to acquire structural data. To record a point, the investigator enters the point code using the CODE BOX, brings the point into best focus using the fine-focus control, and touches the point on the screen with the GRAF/PEN. The first point recorded is used as the origin of the generalized coordinate system for all points. The second point is the location of the soma. Starting at the root of the selected process, points are recorded along the bifurcating structure in the sequential order of the stick model.

As the points are being recorded along a fiber, the continuation of the fiber frequently passes laterally from view on the monitor screen. To continue recording points along the fiber, the investigator finds an easily identifiable point in the tissue, records the point with a CODE 10, translates the microscope stage, and records the same point again with a CODE 10. These points generate lateral translation parameters.

A dendritic or axonal process may not be contained within a single slice of tissue. To continue recording points along a fiber as it passes from one slice of tissue to the next, the investigator presses "S" on the console keyboard to enter the *slice-matching routine*. The last point recorded before entering this routine was located at one surface of the tissue slice. Usually a number of fibers will be seen exiting or entering through the surface near the fiber that is to be continued. The cut end points of a number of these fibers are recorded using the GRAF/PEN. The set is terminated using RETURN on the console keyboard. The pattern of these points is seen on the display scope. The next slice in the series is mounted on the microscope stage and the corresponding surface is brought into focus. Using gross histological observations, the appropriate area can be located. Again the GRAF/PEN is used to record the cut end points of a number of fibers and terminates with a RETURN. The two sets of points and a small "x" are seen on the display scope. The first and second potentiometers on the POT BOX vertically and horizontally translate the second set of points. The third and fourth potentiometers vertically and horizontally translate the "x" cursor. The fifth potentiometer rotates the second set of points using the cursor location as the axis of rotation. When a sufficient number of points match to ensure identification of the continuing fiber and appropriate transformation parameters, the "R" is pressed on the console keyboard. The x and y translation lengths, the x and y rotation axis coordinates, and the rotation angle are stored in two words of the point data array with a CODE 13.

Occasionally the investigator may wish to delete points already recorded. By pressing "E" on the console keyboard, the *erase routine* is entered. The console requests the number of points to be deleted from the end of the point data sequence. The investigator responds by entering the desired number using the console keyboard. The point data array and display array index counters are changed by the appropriate amount and the recording of points can continue as if the deleted point had never been recorded.

All the points that represent the reconstruction of a single neuron are considered as a single structure. The individual processes are treated as substructure. When the investigator completes the recording of points for a process, he presses "F" on the console keyboard to enter the *fiber termination routine*. A separation code is entered in the point data array and the number of points for this process is entered in the associated data array.

When the complete neuron has been reconstructed, the investigator presses

"R" on the console keyboard. The console then requests a file name to be entered on the keyboard. After entry, the contents of the associated cell data array and the point data array are transferred to a DEC tape file for permanent storage. The investigator then presses "M" on the console keyboard to return to the system monitor for data processing.

7. Data Processing

Once the structural data have been collected with A.R.G.O.S., the data are easily edited, transformed, and analyzed using computer data-processing techniques. These techniques are extremely fast, flexible, and accurate. Figure 5 is a schematic diagram of the flow of data through the data-processing computer programs.

The output data of A.R.G.O.S. for each neuron are in a fixed word format. The coordinate points have not been transformed to a generalized system. However, the translation and rotation parameters are included in the structural data sequence.

Program PRINT A prints out the associated cell data and the point data in the fixed word format on the teletype. This program is used primarily to examine the collected data for errors. Frequently, examination of the collected data will reveal errors that can be corrected without remeasuring the neuron.

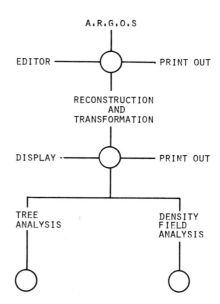

Fig. 5. Data-processing flow diagram.

Program DATA EDITOR is used to manually enter changes into the associated cell data and the point data arrays.

In order to conserve computer core memory space and to preserve the precision of the measurements of the coordinates, the structural data are not transformed by A.R.G.O.S. into a generalized coordinate system. This transformation is performed by program XFORM. The transformed data are stored in a new file on DEC tape in floating-point format. This floating-point format is the proper one for input to FORTRAN computer programs.

Program PRINT B prints out on the teletype the associated cell data and the point data which have been transformed to a generalized coordinate system in floating-point format. This program is also used to check the structural data for errors. Program DISPLAY uses computer graphics techniques to provide a visual presentation of structural data. These techniques will be discussed later in detail.

In general terms, the *FORTRAN analysis* programs extract structural variables from the structural data and analyze the variables using statistical and analytical methods. One of the major objectives of our analysis is to determine which variables are fundamental or useful to the understanding of neuronal structure. This search of variables will entail the development of a large number of computer programs. The advantage of using FORTRAN is apparent in this application. The usual structure of a FORTRAN program is a main routine and several subroutines. The data read-in routines, statistical routines, histogram routines, curve-fitting routines, and plotting routines are written as subroutines called from a main routine. The main routine calculates the variable to be analyzed from the structural data. Frequently, the results of one variable analysis will suggest the examination of another. To select another variable usually requires slight modification of the main routine. Hence many structural variables can be examined with little additional program development.

8. Computer Graphics Display

Computer graphics provides the important link between the quantitative structural data and the classical visual morphology of the histological preparation. By a variety of techniques, computer graphics can visually present a three-dimensional neuronal structure on a CRT screen for study (Lindsay, 1971; Levinthal and Ware, 1972; Selverston, 1973). Rarely can the neurohistologist visualize the complete structure of a neuron since the complete structure is very often contained in a number of serial tissue sections. Computer reconstruction and visual display by means of computer graphics give the classical morphologist a unique and dramatic presentation. This technique has been used to gain valuable information about the classical morphology of neurons not obtainable

solely through the use of the microscope. From a practical point of view, computer graphics has been useful in verifying experimental structural data.

A graphics display program was developed to read the structural data in floating-point format from the tape unit and to display a projected view on the CRT screen. The parameter potentiometers on the panel of the computer are used to change the magnification and to rotate the structure on the screen. The axon and dendrites can be presented individually by pressing the corresponding process number on the console keyboard.

This display program utilizes the point-plot mode of operation; that is, only the data points are intensified on the screen. In practice, the points are close enough together to form a line (see Fig. 6). Rotation or change in magnification of the structure requires lengthy computation. During these operations, the image has an undesirable flickering appearance.

There are other types of computer graphics systems that are more suited to display the structural data collected using A.R.G.O.S. A system using the *vector graphics* mode of display can intensify the line between data points. Some of these systems are available with analog hardware for rotation and change of

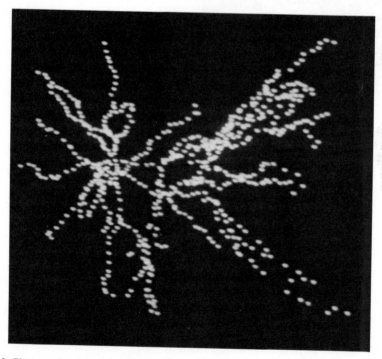

Fig. 6. Photograph of a reconstructed small pyramidal cell on the screen of the display oscilloscope using the point-plot mode.

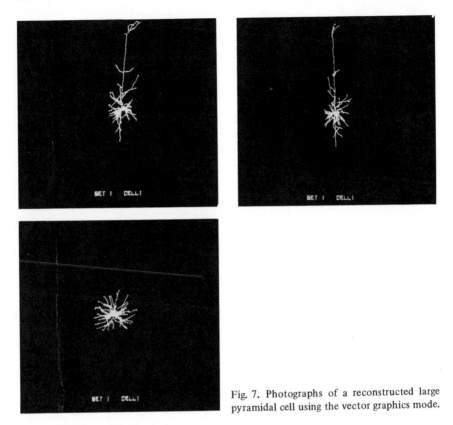

Fig. 7. Photographs of a reconstructed large pyramidal cell using the vector graphics mode.

magnification. Continuous rotation or changes in magnification are accomplished without noticeable flickering. Figure 7 illustrates the use of vector graphics to display the three-dimensional structure of a neuron.

9. *Quantitative Analysis*

There are two general quantitative analysis schemes that have been applied to the structural data collected with this system. Looking through the microscope at a delicately Golgi-impregnated neuron, one is struck with its remarkable similarity of appearance to the arborization of a tree.

The first general analysis scheme is to treat the dendrites and axons as bifurcating treelike structures. The focus of this method is on the individual branches and their position in the topology of the fibrous structure. A number

of structural variables have been calculated from the structural data such as branch lengths and branch angles. Statistical parameters and frequency distributions have been determined for various categories of branch variables. Probability density functions were fitted to the experimental frequency distributions (see Lindsay, Chapter 8).

This method of analysis is useful in the attempt to understand the laws that determine the bifurcating pattern of the neuronal processes. Of particular interest is determination of whether the branching patterns are of a rigid or stochastic structural design.

The second general analysis scheme is to treat the neuronal structure as a fiber density field. In this approach, variables associated with the overall geometry of the neuronal processes are of interest. Variables associated with individual branches are not of concern.

One variable chosen for analysis is the fiber surface area per unit volume in space. The objective is to obtain an analytical function that expresses the average density of fiber surface area at a point in space. In a sense, this scheme smooths the variable over the individual branches of the neuronal processes.

A straightforward method for computation of the surface area density is to divide space into small cubes and calculate the total length of fiber contained in each cube. Using the total length of fiber, an estimated fiber diameter, and the volume of the cube, the surface area per unit volume is easily calculated for each cube. However, there is still left the task of generalizing the cube densities to an analytical density function.

Although this cube density method is straightforward in its application, a more sophisticated technique of three-dimensional Fourier series analysis in rectangular, cylindrical, and spherical coordinate systems has been developed (see Lindsay, Chapter 9). Structural parameters determined using this technique yield quantitative parameters that are easily identified with classical morphological descriptions.

10. Conclusion

Line drawings, prepared with the aid of drawing tubes attached to the microscope, have been the principal medium in the study of neuronal structure. However, these drawings represent only a projected view of the structure and do not contain its tridimensional aspect. Mannen (1966, 1975) has developed a clever and esthetically pleasing tridimensional photographic technique for the graphic reconstruction of the soma and its processes. These techniques require a large effort by a skilled morphologist and the product is a graphic representation, a form still requiring transformation for quantitative analysis.

Data models have been developed for the numerical representation of neuronal structure. This type of structural representation requires a large amount of data. A semiautomated data-acquisition system has been discussed in detail which uses commercially available hardware components. A software operating system has been developed to assist and guide the investigator with the measuring procedure. Modern data-processing techniques have been used from the collection of data to the final product of the analysis.

The development of data-acquisition systems for the quantitative reconstruction of neuronal structures arms the neuroscientist with a new and powerful tool to attack the structure of nervous systems.

ACKNOWLEDGMENTS

The support and the encouragement of the Scheibels have been greatly appreciated. Research by the author was supported by USPHS Grant NS 10657, N.I.N.D.S. The assistance and encouragement of my wife, Barbara, in the preparation of this chapter are gratefully acknowledged.

11. References

Davenport, H. A., 1960, *Histological and Histochemical Techniques*, Saunders, Philadelphia.

Garvey, C., Young, J., Coleman, P., and Simon, W., 1973, Automated three-dimensional dendrite tracking system, *Electroencephalogr. and Clin. Neurophysiol.* 35:199–204.

Harth, E. M., and Lindsay, R. D., 1968, *Connectivity of the Cerebral Cortex: A Computerized Study*, Office of Naval Research Final Report, March 22.

Ledley, R. S., 1964, High-speed automatic analysis of biomedical pictures, *Science* 146:216–222.

Levinthal, C., and Ware, R., 1972, Three-dimensional reconstruction from serial sections, *Nature (London)* 236:207–210.

Lindsay, R. D., 1971, Connectivity of the cerebral cortex, dissertation, Physics Department, Syracuse University.

Mannen, H., 1966, Contribution to the quantitative study of nervous tissue: A new method for measurement of the volume and surface area of neurons, *J. Comp. Neurol.* 126:75–90.

Mannan, H., 1975, Reconstruction of axonal trajectory of individual neurons in the spinal cord using Golgi-stained serial sections, *J. Comp. Neurol.* 159:357–374.

McManus, J. F., and Mowry, R. W., 1960, *Staining Methods Histological and Histochemical*, Hoeber, New York.

Ramon-Moliner, E., 1957, A chlorate-formaldehyde modification of the Golgi method, *Stain Technol.* 32:105–116.

Reddy, D., Davis, E., Ohlander, R., and Bihary, D., 1973, Computer analysis of neuronal structure, in: *Intracellular Staining in Neurobiology* (S. B. Kater and C. Nicholson, eds.), Springer-Verlag, New York.

Selverston, A., 1973, The use of intracellular dye injections in the small neural network, in: *Intracellular Staining in Neurobiology* (S. B. Kater and C. Nicholson, eds.), Springer-Verlag, New York.

Sholl, D. A., 1956, *The Organization of the Cerebral Cortex*, Methuen, London.

Wann, D., Woolsey, T., Dierker, M., and Cowan, W. M., 1973, An on-line digital-computer system for the semiautomatic analysis of Golgi-impregnated neurons, *IEEE Trans. Biomed. Eng.* **20**:233−248.

2

Computer Reconstruction of Invertebrate Nerve Cells

Sheryl Glasser, John Miller, N. G. Xuong, and Allen Selverston

1. Introduction

The use of computer graphics as an aid in the study of nerve cell architecture has become increasingly useful. Computer displays can serve not only to visualize the three-dimensional structure of neurons but also to quantify their important anatomical parameters. The ease with which such measurements can be made provides a new and important tool to those of us hoping to correlate the structure of single and identifiable nerve cells with their functional properties and development. We are in a position to make such correlations in our laboratory with a fair degree of precision for two reasons. The first is that we use invertebrate preparations in which we can identify specific cells and return to them repeatedly. The second is the great advance made in the techniques of intracellular staining. Once electrophysiological measurements have been made, identifiable neurons can be selectively stained for cytoarchitectural studies at both the light and electron microscopic levels.

A great deal of useful information can be obtained by simply looking at serial sections or whole mounts of such selectively stained preparations. However, the information content of such material can be increased markedly by computer analysis.

Basically, the problems involved in the reconstruction process are familiar to anyone who has worked with computer graphics. The structure must first be digitized: by assigning x, y, and z coordinates to its parts, the vectors which produce the image can be displayed on some kind of cathode-ray terminal

Sheryl Glasser, John Miller, N. G. Xuong, and Allen Selverston · Department of Biology, University of California San Diego, La Jolla, California 92093.

(CRT), the end product being a reproduction of the three-dimensional features of the object under investigation. Once this has been accomplished, programs must be written to make the appropriate measurements and to manipulate the image in ways useful to the investigator.

There are many methods to accomplish these goals with the varieties of hardware presently available. In general, the greater the investment in hardware the less software development is necessary. We shall describe in detail the system we have arrived at after some 4 years of experience, the reasons we made the hardware and software choices we did, and the purposes to which we are applying them.

To a large extent, our procedures followed naturally from the histological methods we had been using. These methods basically consisted of injecting neurons with the fluorescent dye Procion yellow after they had been examined physiologically. More recently, we have been injecting dyes which can be seen in both the light and electron microscope. We will consider separately the procedures for reconstructing images from each of these levels of resolution.

Neurons in the stomatogastric ganglion of the lobster are identified by correlating the intracellular soma activity with extracellularly recorded spikes in the identified motor nerves. If the neurons are not spontaneously active, they can be fired by passage of current into the somata. This produces a spike in the peripheral axon. Alternatively, the axon can be fired antidromically and an attenuated spike recorded from the cell body. A diagrammatic sketch of cell positions is made as the neurons are identified so that they can be returned to at the end of the experiment and injected with dye.

At the light microscopic level, the procedure for the complete reconstruction of a neuron is organized as follows: (1) injection of fluorescent dye into an identified neuron of the ganglion (the structure containing the cells); (2) fixation, dehydration, and clearing of the ganglion; (3) embedding and sectioning of the ganglion; (4) color photography of each section; (5) digitization of all fluorescent images on the photographs; (6) alignment of the digitized section images; and (7) connection of corresponding contours in adjacent section images to form a reconstructed image of the cell.

The hardware we use in the computer-aided steps of this procedure consists of a PDP-11/45 computer, an acoustic digitizing tablet, a 35-mm slide projector, and a Vector General interactive graphics terminal. The software was written largely in FORTRAN, and relies heavily on the FORTRAN-callable subroutines of a version of GIGL (general interactive graphics language) developed especially for the Vector General–PDP-11 system.

Our procedure for the three-dimensional reconstruction of serial electron micrographs is essentially the same as that for light micrographs except that the programming for the connection of the profiles has been modified. These programs will be described in detail in a subsequent section.

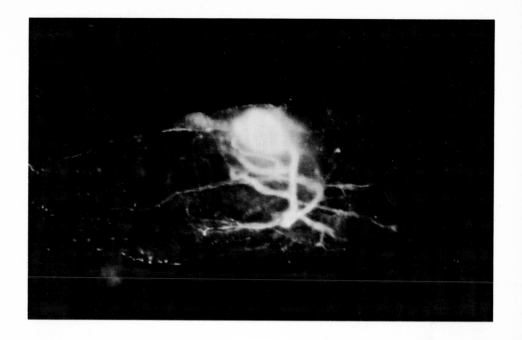

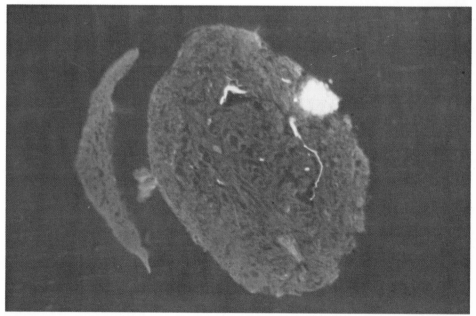

Fig. 1. A Procion-yellow-filled pyloric dilator neuron (PD cell) is shown in a whole mount of the ganglion (upper). A cross-section 10 μm thick made from the same ganglion shows the fluorescent profiles of the injected neuron (lower).

2. Procedure

The methods used in dye injection and histology depend on the particular dye to be used, and have been described in great detail elsewhere (Selverston, 1973). For reconstructions at the light microscopic level, we have chosen the fluorescent dye Procion yellow (M4RS or M4RAN). This dye is injected directly into the cell body (soma) of the neuron through a glass capillary microelectrode. The dye may be introduced into the cell either by pressure injection or, since the dye is charged, by passing current through the electrode (iontophoresis). The latter method uses the Procion dye ions as the actual charge carriers, and is the method we most frequently use in our work.

After sufficient time for dye migration has elapsed, about 12 hr, the ganglion is fixed, dehydrated in alcohol, and cleared in methylbenzoate. When fixed, cleared properly, and illuminated with near-ultraviolet light, the Procion-filled cell fluoresces a brilliant yellow against the dim green background fluorescence of the unstained tissue (Fig. 1a).

After the whole mount has been photographed from several angles, the ganglion is embedded in paraffin and serially sectioned at 10 μm. It is extremely important not to lose any of the sections at this stage, since a sequential reconstruction would be faulty with any sections missing. The sections are mounted sequentially in rows on a microscope slide, and when viewed with ultraviolet illumination appear as in Fig. 1b.

Here the particular advantage of Procion yellow dye injection over other techniques such as cobalt staining and the Golgi method becomes obvious. The latter two stains do not fluoresce, but simply increase the optical density of the stained cell, making it black against a translucent background. When such preparations are viewed in cross-section at high power, any dark spots in unstained areas of the ganglion could be mistaken for small processes of a stained neuron and confuse the reconstruction process. The added cue of color contrast between a Procion-filled cell and its background makes such mistakes much less likely. In addition, the Procion staining is specific; that is, one knows in advance which cell is being stained.

The only major disadvantage of Procion yellow is that it cannot be used efficiently to resolve the finest order of neuronal processes (those of 0.5 μm or less). Even if it could be assumed that these finest processes are completely filled, two problems would remain. First, the dimensions of these processes are at the limits of resolution of regular light microscopy. Since Procion yellow is not electron dense, it is extremely difficult to trace the process through serial electron micrographs (Purves and McMahon, 1972). Second, since the visibility of Procion-filled processes depends on fluorescent radiation rather than on absorption of light, the brightness of a Procion-filled process will depend on the amount of Procion it contains and thus on its diameter. Long photographic exposure times are usually necessary to bring out the finest processes, but this has not been a severe problem in our work since stomatogastric cells do not appear to have a significant number of processes with diameter less than $0.5-1$ μm. The optimum section thickness seems to be about 10 μm, since (1) in thicker sections the background fluorescence begins to obscure the detail of the finest processes and (2) thinner sections necessitate longer photographic exposure times to bring out the Procion-filled contours. Also, the thinner the sections, the greater the amount of core memory space needed in the later computer-assisted steps of the reconstruction.

Photography of the sections is done using a Zeiss universal photomicroscope. Sections are illuminated with ultraviolet light passed through a BG12 exciter filter (peak transmission at 400 nm) and spectrally sharpened with an FITC 490-nm interference filter. The latter filter sharpens the spectral transmission range of the ultraviolet illuminating beam, minimizing unwanted background fluorescence of the unstained tissue. A 35-mm color slide is taken of each section through two barrier filters. A 530-nm filter selects for the yellow fluorescence, and a 470-nm filter cuts out the intrinsic fluorescence of the 530-nm filter.

The subsequent steps of the reconstruction are all carried out with the aid of the computer and, as previously noted, involve digitizing, aligning, and connecting the photographed fluorescent images. Before discussion of these last stages of the reconstruction, a complete description of the computer hardware and its configuration is in order.

3. Hardware

The system on which the reconstructions are performed consists of (1) a PDP-11/45 computer with teletype, DECtape, and magnetic disk; (2) an acoustic data tablet and 35-mm slide projector; and (3) a Vector General interactive graphics display terminal. A block diagram and photograph of the system are shown in Fig. 2.

3.1. Computer

The PDP-11/45 computer (Digital Equipment Corp., Maynard, Mass.) used in our studies is operated with 32 K of core memory, two magnetic disk drives, two DECtape drives, and fast floating-point hardware. It has a 16-bit word structure and an average cycle time of about 500 nsec. Systems programs allow full FORTRAN IV capability, as well as Basic and the PDP-11 Macro assembly

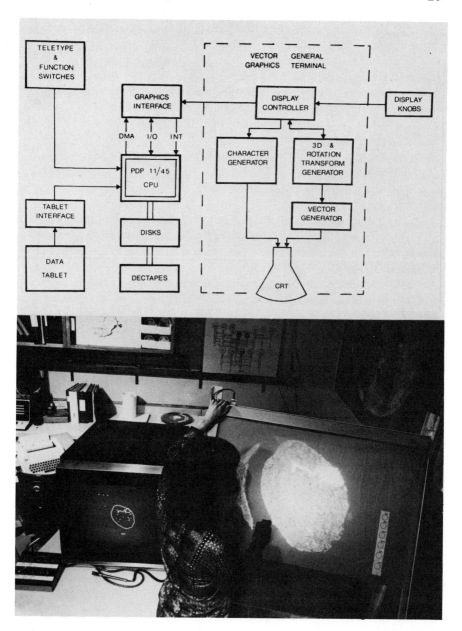

Fig. 2. Block diagram of the computer graphics system we use for the reconstruction of dye-filled neurons. The lower photo shows the interactive process of tracing out the profiles and ganglionic outline on a data tablet. Color slides of serial sections are projected from the rear of the tablet.

language. Programs are entered on the teletype through an editing program and can be stored along with data on the disks (1.2 M words capacity) or on DECtapes (225 K words capacity). An additional routine has been written which enables the teletype keyboard to be treated as a peripheral "switch box." In this mode, an interrupt is generated every time the keyboard is hit, allowing any key to act as a spring-mounted switch associated with various program functions. The use of such a versatile switch box is necessary in several of our reconstruction programs.

3.2. Digitizing Equipment

The initial step of the digitization procedure can take place either with the whole mounts or with sectioned tissue. Because we are interested in the accurate determination of process diameters, we work with the sectioned neurons (for techniques of digitizing whole mounts, see Wann *et al.*, 1973).

At this point, it is important to digress about how images such as sectioned profiles or particular portions of an electron micrograph could be entered into a computer. It is possible, at least in theory, to have some device such as a TV camera scan a picture and differentiate the boundaries of those portions which are relevant from those which are irrelevant. If the picture is simple enough – e.g., black chromosomes on a white background – a pattern-recognition algorithm can recognize the edges of the chromosomes from a videcon scanner with a high degree of fidelity. But if there are irrelevant structures which have a similar appearance to the structures of interest, the problem of pattern recognition becomes increasingly complex. The great advantage of such automatic scanning is speed, but it would require a very powerful and expensive computer with a large core memory together with many years of manpower to develop the software for pattern recognition. Since we did not wish to devote our time to the pattern-recognition problem but instead to the structural analysis of nerve cells, we, as most others, opted for digitizing all relevant material, fluorescent profiles or parts of electron micrographs, by hand. We adopted an interactive process in which the brain of the operator is used as the pattern-recognition device and the computer as a notebook. The computer displays the profiles as they are being entered by the operator, allowing him to detect and correct any mistake.

For digitization of the visual images, we selected a large (36- by 36-inch) acoustic data tablet; its size gives good resolution and it is translucent, so that serial sections for an entire neuron can be put onto 35-mm slides and projected sequentially from the rear. As each slide is projected, the boundary of the ganglion and the profiles of the injected cell or cells are quickly and accurately digitized by a trained operator using a minimal number of points. The data tablet (GRAF/PEN by Science Accessories Corp., Southport, Conn.) consists of a flat plastic surface with strip microphones along two edges. An electric stylus emits a sonic pulse whenever its tip touches the tablet. A control unit interprets the responses from the sensors as x, y coordinates by comparing their time of arrival with the time of generation of the pulse. These coordinates are transmitted to the computer and the contours are displayed on the graphics terminal as they are traced out.

The coordinates are digitized to 10-bit accuracy, giving a resolution of about 1.0 mm on the tablet. Repeated digitization of a single point on the tablet gave a measurement with standard deviation of 0.84 bit on each axis, equivalent to a total standard deviation in each coordinate position of 1.0 mm. This represents approximately 0.5 μm on our photographic image, a resolution comparable to that of the photograph itself.

The color photographs of the ganglion sections are rear-projected onto the tablet by a Kodak model 860 carousel projector with a 2½-inch f/3.5 Ektanar lens. The tablet and projector are mounted on specially built racks to keep the projection beam perpendicular to the plane of the tablet. In setting up the equipment for digitization, the minimum noticeable displacement and rotation of the projector from its normal position were 2 mm and 3°, respectively. Some deviation in the positions of individual slides falling into the projector may also exist. To test the effect of these deviations on the final digitized image, a slide of a grid was repeatedly digitized with the various deviations set at all possible combinations of their maximal values. The worse-case error in image scale was found to be less than 0.2% along each axis.

Several other methods that were tried and found to be impractical or inaccurate, including a rotating-drum digitizer in conjunction with a computer-driven cursor, have been described elsewhere (Selverston, 1973).

3.3. Graphics Display System

An essential component of any system developed for the purpose of reconstruction is some means for visualization of the final reconstructed image. The output device used could be a simple line plotter, if (1) the image does not need to be rotated in real time to aid visualization and (2) the alignment can be done automatically without any operator interaction. *Neither* of these conditions is met in our case, however. The images are very complex, incorporating up to 1500 vectors, so that a hard copy line plot alone is too slow. The ability to rotate the image in real time about all three axes is extremely helpful in properly visualizing such an image. Finally, the decision to rely on operator judgment rather than automated pattern recognition means that constant monitoring and control of the reconstruction procedure are required.

With these factors in mind, the obvious choice for graphic output is some type of CRT display device. Three possible alternatives exist: a storage oscilloscope, a raster-scanning video terminal, or an interactive refresh-type graphics device. For our purposes, the first two alternatives were unacceptable. No video terminal exists with line resolution comparable to the resolution of our data. And although an image can be displayed at all possible angles on a storage scope, it cannot be rotated in real time. Reconstructions were successfully performed by this laboratory using a storage scope and a CalComp plotter, but the process was excessively time consuming, and it was necessary to make a movie to visualize the reconstructed figure in three dimensions.

The device we use is a Vector General (VG) real-time interactive graphics display terminal (Vector General Co., Canoga Park, Calif.), with the operations of rotation and translation performed directly by hardware. The actual values of these parameters are controlled by the operator through a set of dials (hereafter called the *display knobs*) associated with the display terminal. The VG has its own high-speed processor, and uses one direct memory access (DMA) line, one programmed input—output channel, and one interrupt level of the host computer. The image is created by setting up a "display list" of coordinates in the host computer's core memory, which is scanned by the VG's processor through the DMA line.

The large 13- by 14-inch screen is easily photographed with both still and movie cameras. Photographic stereo pairs may be made from any viewing angle. When the picture contains two or more separate images which can be displayed independently (e.g., reconstructions of two cells having synaptic contacts or the pre- and postsynaptic sides of a synapse), a multicolor photograph can be obtained by multiple exposures of the two images through different color filters on the same frame of color film. Examples are shown later in the chapter.

The configuration of the complete hardware system described above was arrived at after experimentation with various other digitizing and display devices (Fig 2). The system seems optimal for several reasons. First, we have tried to minimize the cost of the system by eliminating excess-automation "overkill." Examples of covenient optional features that can be obtained on Vector General or comparable graphics terminals but are not necessary for studies such as ours include picture perspective, hidden-line suppression, and circular arc generation. On the other hand, options such as extrashort-persistency tube phosphor have been found to be worth the extra cost. Second, the above system is truly *interactive* in that it maximizes the dependence on operator judgment rather than automated pattern-recognition algorithms at critical levels of decision making.

Many of the decisions we have made, both on hardware configuration and on software development, have depended on our need to measure process diameters in addition to length and connectivity. This greatly increases the amount of core memory necessary over that needed for the generation of simple stick figures. Depending on the particular goals of the research project, various modifications of our system might be considered. If simpler structures are to be reconstructed, a PDP-11/05 processor could be substituted fairly easily for our 11/45. The processors for the two machines are essentially the same, except that the 11/05 is slower. A DECtape operating system can replace the disk system where speed and storage capacity are not crucial factors. Where image resolution is not as critical, smaller data tablets and/or video terminals might be substituted.

4. Software

The stages involved in the computer reconstruction procedure are (1) digitization of the information in the sections, (2) alignment of the sections with respect to one another, (3) computation of the center point and diameter of each contour, (4) connection of the contours into a stick figure, and (5) reordering and indexing of the branching pattern topologically. Steps (1), (2), and (4) require operator interaction; (3) and (5) are automatic.

The programming for all of the steps below relies on a library of FORTRAN-callable subroutines called GIGL (general interactive graphics language). GIGL was developed originally for the PDP-10, LDS-1 system at Princeton University and modified to run on our present system.* These subroutines form a software interface between the programmer and the processor of the graphics terminal, which can understand only a restricted set of machine language commands. To draw a vector, for example, a programmer need only make two calls to GIGL subroutines: CALL POS (X1, Y1, Z1) to position the beam at the beginning of the vector and CALL DRAWT (X2, Y2, Z2) to connect the beginning and end points of the vector. It should be noted that although the general software scheme described below could be copied for many other hardware systems having FORTRAN capabilities, the specific calling sequences and data word structure used will be dependent on the particular graphics system and FORTRAN libraries used.

---

*GIGL was developed for the PDP-10, LDS-1 system at Princeton by W. T. Wipke and T. M. Dyott and modified for the 11–45 system by Sheryl Glasser. The latter version is available from A. I. Selverston.

4.1. Digitization

As described above, color slides of the ganglion sections are rear-projected onto the data tablet for digitization. Average diameter of the projected section image is about 2 ft, making the image scale approximately 2 cm per 10 μm on the original section. The fluorescent processes in each section show up in three forms: (1) tiny spots (diameter less than 2 mm) digitized as two points on the circumference representing the diameter, (2) long skinny contours (width less than 2 mm) digitized as "open" contours by sampling several points along the center line and two points across the width to represent the process diameter, and (3) large spots or irregularly shaped contours for the wall of the ganglion and nonfluorescent somata which may appear in the section. These are digitized as cues for later section alignment (see Fig. 3b).

As the contours are traced out with the electric stylus, a "display list" of coordinates is created in the central processor's core memory and displayed on the graphics terminal simultaneously, enabling the operator to see what has already been entered. There are two arrays created along with the display list: an index list containing a nonzero entry for each fluorescent contour and a zero entry for each wall cue, and a diameter list containing the measured values for diameters of open contours. Diameters of closed contours are calculated in a later program.

The program begins by initializing a "menu," or list of commands from which selections are to be made on the data tablet. A printed menu, consisting of a strip of paper with five small circles drawn on it, is taped to the extreme right-hand side of the tablet. A menu item is selected whenever the stylus is touched to the tablet within one of these circles. A menu selection simply sets a flag, and the next nonmenu point is processed and indexed depending on the value of the flag.

The menu items are

WALL: Indicates that the next points entered will represent a non-fluorescent contour to be used for alignment purposes. A zero is entered in the index list.

NEW: Indicates that next points entered will represent a fluorescent open or closed contour or will be two points representing a tiny spot. An index number is entered in the index list.

DIAM: Indicates that next two points entered are to be taken as a diameter measurement whose value holds for every point of the last, presumably open, contour. A nonzero value is entered in the index and diameter lists.

ERASE: Deletes the last digitized contour.

END: Causes the digitized information to be stored on the disk and prepares the program to accept another section film.

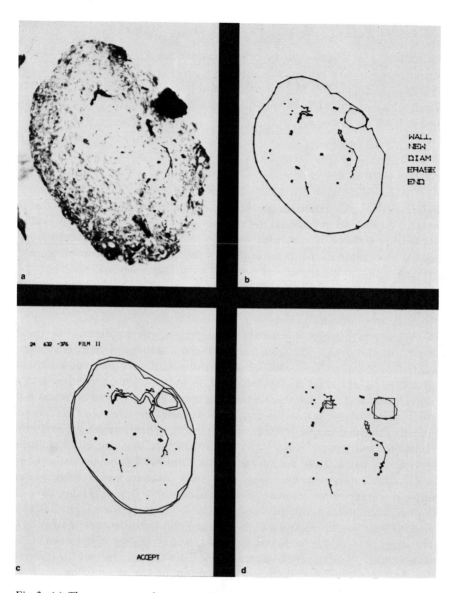

Fig. 3. (a) The appearance of a cross-section through a ganglion with the processes of the injected cell visible as black profiles. (b) The same section displayed on the screen of the graphics terminal after digitization. (c) Two sequential sections after manual alignment. (d) The first section (b) with wall trees removed and with computed center points and diameters of the profiles represented as squares.

The operator proceeds with the digitizing, one section at a time, referencing the original ganglion section on the microscope when there is doubt about any detail. When all slides have been digitized, a photograph of a micrometer slide is projected onto the tablet, and the distance corresponding to the section thickness is digitized. The data from each section are stored in three disk blocks, totaling 768 16-bit words, divided into 512 display list elements and 256 words for indexing information. Data files are stored in a contiguous master file.

4.2. Alignment

A major decision that had to be made was whether to align the sections before or after digitization. A serious problem with biological material is that it is often difficult to put fiducial marks onto sections, and one must rely on the continuous features of the tissue itself to secure accurate alignment of one section with another. It is possible to align each section prior to photography, yielding a film strip in which all sections are in alignment and need only be projected and digitized (Ware, 1972). However, we again picked what seemed to us the easiest procedure, aligning the sections after they had been digitized and stored in the computer.

An initial attempt at achieving the alignment with a program that would search for the orientations giving the maximum amount of overlap between adjacent sections was unsuccessful because many small spots may not overlap at all due to the thickness of the sectioning. In addition, the program took very much longer than the same procedure performed by an operator. We did not pursue this problem further but may do so at some later time if a faster, more accurate algorithm can be devised. Our alignment method utilizes the hardware translation and rotation capabilities of the graphics terminal, although such movements were initially accomplished with software. Two sequential sections at a time are displayed on the screen. The display knobs are used to translate and rotate the image of the second film with respect to the first until attainment of (1) maximum overlap of the large contours, (2) lining up of long skinny processes, and (3) superposition of the ganglion wall and other cues (see Fig. 3c). The values obtained for the necessary translation and rotation of the second film are then used to create a new display list for the contours. This new list replaces the old list on the disk storage. The contours of the second film are now displayed as stationary and those of the next film read in as the movable one.

Here again, as in the digitizing program, the original microscope slides are referred to if any doubt exists about exact alignment.

4.3. Computation of Contour Centers and Diameters

After alignment, the section information is put in the data format that will be used for reconstruction. The serial number of the preparation, type of cell, and date are logged officially into an identification array as the computer requests them. The computer also requests the number of sections and the record where the digitized micrometer measurement is stored. From this information it computes the section thickness in tablet coordinates. A "phony" thickness is computed from the number of sections, which is used only during the reconstruction so that the entire cell can be displayed within the allowed range $Z = \pm 2047$ without shrinking the section size. The identification array, number of sections, and the two thickness values are added to the identification file.

Next, the sections are automatically read in and displayed one at a time. The wall cues are removed, so that the display-list maximum length is reduced from 512 to 420 words. Then center point coordinates and diameter are computed for each process and stored in an array, hereafter referred to as the *POINT array*, as follows. For a long skinny process, i.e., an open contour with a nonzero value in the diameter array, the coordinates of each point of the contour are stored in the point array together with its measured width as a diameter value. For a contour consisting of only two points and having the value zero in the diameter array, the midpoint of the line joining the two points is stored as the center, and the diameter is taken as the length of the line. Finally, a contour with more than two points but with a zero-diameter entry is taken to be a closed contour. Its center point and diameter are computed by fitting the contour with rectangles oriented at different angles and choosing the rectangle whose area is a minimum. The center of the rectangle is used as the center of the contour, and the diameter is given as the width of the rectangle (see Fig. 3d). The reasoning behind this criterion is that a contour that appears as an elliptical process is actually a process of circular cross-section intersecting the plane of the section at an angle. The diameter of such a process would be the semi-minor axis of the ellipse.

The POINT array for each section consists of 348 words. Of these, 345 are allocated for up to 115 triplets specifying the diameter and center (x, y) coordinates of each contour. The remaining three words specify (1) the total number of points in the section, (2) the Z-axis position of the section measured in the phony Z thickness units, and (3) a value of $Z + \frac{1}{2}\Delta Z$, where ΔZ is the phony thickness. This last value allows for new points to be later added to the list halfway between two sections.

4.4. Connection of Digitized Contours

The aim of the connection program is to join together the points contained in the POINT array into a three-dimensional stick figure which, since each point has an associated diameter measurement, represents a tree of sequential cylindrical segments.

Two types of output are generated by this program. The first type consists of changes in the POINT array: additions, deletions, and modifications to any diameter assignments and point positions that are obviously in error because of faulty "judgment" by the algorithms which made those assignments. The second type of output generated is the display list (the *STICK array*) for the stick figure, created by connecting the contours in the POINT list. The program displays the contours for up to three sections at a time. The information stored in the POINT array is also displayed for each section, as squares superimposed on their corresponding contours, just as in Fig. 3d. The ensemble can be rotated around the vertical axis to be seen from any angle. The operator observes the display, corrects any obvious errors made in the POINT list, and connects the

Table I. CONNEC Operation Features

Flags				Switches
/F	Films (enter 215 format)		9	Advance film
			0	Back up film
/G	Gain			
/NG	No gain	/C	1	Connect
		/A	2	Delete last connection
			3	Indicates next 1 = move
/S	Squares			
/NS	No squares			
		/P	1	Get center and two diameters
/W	Window		2	Delete point near cursor
/NW	No window		3	Next 1 gets diameter near cursor
/O	Soma	/D	1	Get vector
/Q	Processes	/B	1	Mark near cursor
/NO	Processes		2	Remove mark near cursor
/C	Connect using cursor			
/A	Connect automatically			
/P	New point			
/D	Delete a vector			
/B	Mark branch			
/H	Help			
/K	Store data (kill)			

contours together using the display knobs and the keyboard, which is used as a "switch box" and interrupt device. A brief summary of keyboard interrupt commands is given in Table I.

4.4.1. POINT Correction (/P Mode)

The points computed automatically by the previous program (POINT computation program) are not always optimal. For example, large, curved closed contours are represented automatically as one center point with a large diameter. Such a contour actually represents a longitudinal section through a long process, and the one center point should be replaced by several points along the curve having smaller diameters, as shown in Fig. 4. There are also places where an additional point midway between two sections is desirable. To make such corrections, the section or sections of interest are blown up using a software "zoom" gain until the desired area fills the screen. To add a point, a small "cursor" mark, also displayed on the screen and movable by three display knobs, is moved to the desired location of the new point and a switch is hit. Then the cursor is moved again to two representative points (not necessarily surrounding the new center point), such that the distance between them is the desired diameter of the point, and a switch is hit for each one. It is also possible to copy the diameter of the point nearest the cursor. To delete a point, another switch is hit, and the point nearest the cursor is removed from the list. These operations affect only the POINT list.

4.4.2. Construction of STICK Array (/C or /A Mode)

There are two ways to trace out the stick figure. In the /C mode (cursor), the operator moves the cursor from point to point, and when the appropriate switch is hit, the point nearest the cursor is entered on the list as a "move" or "draw" (i.e., the beam of the display terminal is repositioned, or is swept to the next point, tracing out a vector). In the /A mode (automatic), a distance-minimizing algorithm searches for the next point to be connected. This routine searches for the nearest point to the last point connected that is not within a backwards cone of half-angle 45°. The operator can accept or reject this new connection. If it is rejected, the computer will try the next nearest point, and so on until the correct point is chosen.

The general procedure in making connections is to begin by connecting the soma, which can have contours in up to 15 sections, into an irregular solid roughly elliptical in shape. Then a point is created, if necessary, overlapping the soma for the beginning of the process which leaves it. This main process, which becomes the motor axon, is traced out until it leaves the ganglion. As it is traced out, branches encountered along the way can be marked by using the "/B" switch. This simply displays the letter "B" at the point nearest the cursor when the switch is hit, for the operator's convenience in locating the branch point later on. After constructing the main branch, or at least a piece of it, the operator is free to connect other branches in any order, and in as many pieces as he pleases. Figure 5 shows a cell in the process of being reconstructed.

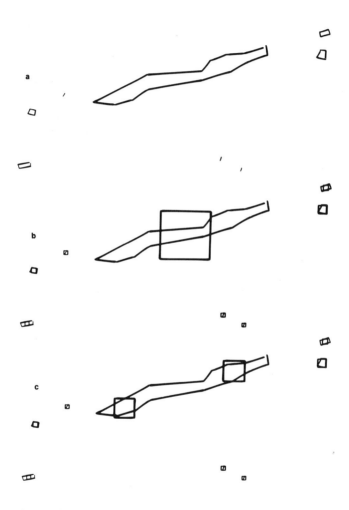

Fig. 4. (a) Output from TABLET including a long closed contour representing a longitudinal section through a fat process. (b) Output from PAKSEC demonstrating inaccurate assignment of diameter. (c) Output from CONNEC demonstrating manual correction of this mistake.

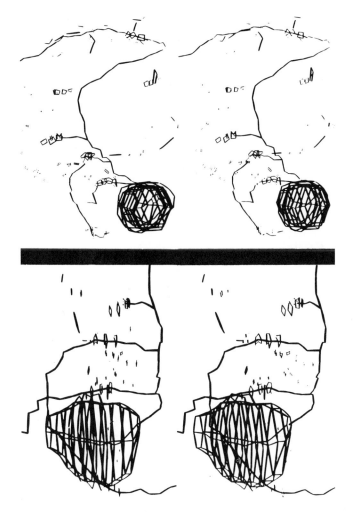

Fig. 5. Stereo pairs of a partially reconstructed cell and profiles from three sections. The cell is displayed from two angles.

4.5. Ordering

The reconstructed neuron is now represented by the STICK display list as a sequence of x, y, z coordinates with a "move" or "draw" instruction for each point, but the branches may be in pieces that are not arranged in any systematic order. The next stage is to transform this list into a sequential representation based on the topological structure, from the soma through primary processes to distal processes. This indexing step is performed automatically by the computer using a topological search on the STICK list. The output consists of (1) four *COORDINATE arrays* for the vertex points $(x, y, z$ and diameter), (2) a *SEGMENT array* which links the points together into segments between branch points, (3) an *ORDER array* which defines the ordering of the segments out from the soma of the neurons, and (4) a *FROM array* which specifies the parent of each daughter segment. For simple applications, the SEGMENT array and the ORDER array may seem redundant, but they are convenient later on when the mathematical modeling procedure may require reordering.

The four COORDINATE arrays $(x, y, z$ diameter) of the vertex points of the tree are created by taking x, y, z of the point in the STICK list and by searching for each corresponding diameter in the POINT list for the appropriate section.

The SEGMENT array, which links the vertex points together into segments, consists simply of a string of the indices of the COORDINATE arrays in sequence. The beginning of each segment is indicated by a negative index value. The program defines a segment as a sequence of points between two consecutive branch points or between a branch point and a terminal point.

Once the SEGMENT array has been constructed, it is necessary to order the segments out from the soma using topological considerations. The first segment, i.e., the big process leaving the soma, is found by testing the first point of each segment for the one which overlaps with one of the soma cross-sections. This segment number is entered on the ORDER list. Since this segment terminates at the first branch point, two or more segments will begin there. The program searches for the next segment via the SEGMENT array by comparing the index of the last point of the previous segment with the indices of the first and last points of all other segments and choosing the first one with the same index. If the newly matched point is the last point of a segment, then the segment was reconstructed in reverse order, i.e., toward the soma instead of away from it; so the program converts the order of the segment immediately. If the segment was reconstructed in pieces, the SEGMENT array is changed to put the pieces together. The program then seeks a segment to attach to the end of the second segment, and so on. As each segment is added to the ORDER list, an addition is made to the FROM list telling what segment it comes from. After the first process has been completed, the program returns to the first segment and looks for all secondary processes out from its end, then all secondary processes branching out from the end of the second segment of the primary processes, and continues until the entire tree is done.

4.6. Display

The reconstructed cell can be displayed in three modes: (1) as a stick figure, which simply shows the processes as a series of lines without diameter information; (2) as a "fat" figure, in which the diameters of the processes are also shown; (3) and as a two-dimensional schematic figure.

4.6.1. Stick Figure

The display list of the stick figure simply consists of points from the COORDINATE array joined together in the proper order, with the soma represented as hexagons connected at the vertices.

4.6.2. Fat Figure

An algorithm has been developed which enables the reconstructed tree to be displayed on a line-drawing system incorporating the proper diameter information so as to suggest the joined cylinders of the model (see Fig. 6). Each tapered cylinder is drawn as four lines (rectangular solid) whose end-point coordinates are determined by setting up little squares of the correct size around each vertex and orienting them perpendicular to the direction of the cylinder axis. The orientation which correctly aligns the squares without twisting them with respect to each other is computed through a complex matrix transformation on the coordinates of each square (see Section 7.1 for more detail).

4.6.3. Two-Dimensional Schematic

The final type of display represents the reconstructed tree in a way that clearly shows its topological structure: number of branches and their placement, diameters, and lengths. This schematic figure appears as a two-dimensional arborization whose branches follow straight lines or straight lines with one bend in them and show proportionally the correct thickness. Such a representation makes it possible to compare the architecture of identified cells of the same type from animal to animal. Because the branching pattern is not necessarily consistent, the program is set up to allow the operator to manipulate the angles of the displayed branches so as to bring out all recognizable features. The algorithm is more fully described in Section 7.2. Figure 7 shows the final schematized reconstruction of the cell pictured in other figures along with the whole mount and three-dimensional reconstruction for comparison.

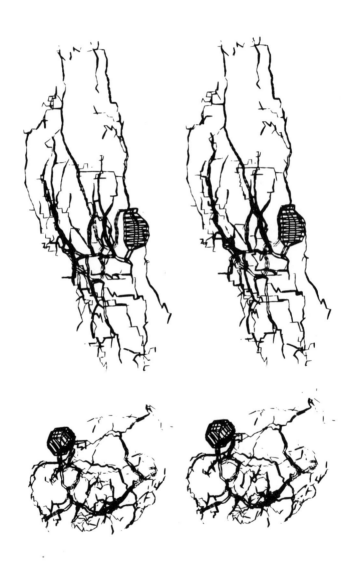

Fig. 6. Stereo pairs of a fully reconstructed cell displayed with diameter information.

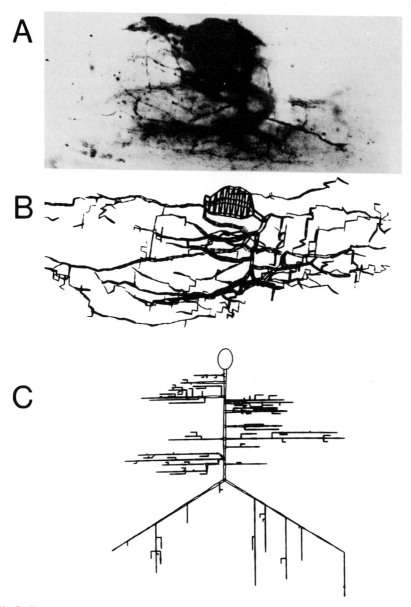

Fig. 7. Computer reconstruction of a pyloric dilator neuron. (A) Procion-yellow-filled whole mount. (B) Three-dimensional reconstruction. (C) Two-dimensional schematic representation of the same cell. From Selverston *et al.* (1976).

5. Prospective Studies

Our original intent in developing a graphics capability for the analysis of neuronal structure was to be able to visualize selectively stained, identifiable neurons as completely as possible. Viewing neurons from a variety of angles discloses a great deal about the general arrangement and complexity of the branching processes. For example, in some cases the processes were arranged along a single plane while in others the processes were arranged more diffusely throughout the neuropil region of the ganglion. One is able, also, to obtain an immediate impression of the gross architectural features of the neuron such as whether it is composed mainly of large- or small-diameter processes, whether the extent of branching is great or small, whether there are many terminal spines on the processes or not. We also hoped to obtain data about the constancy of geometries in identical cells of different animals. We had reason to believe that in our preparation, the lobster stomatogastric ganglion, the three-dimensional form might be variable because the positions of the neuron cell bodies are inconsistent from animal to animal. However, the physiological relationships between these cells are remarkably constant, with each cell having a rather narrowly defined functional role. In considering how such functional reproducibility might be obtained in the light of structural differences, one can postulate a two-dimensional invariance in branch length and node position which would imply electrical constancy despite differences in three-dimensional form. The interactive program, SCHEMA, produces a two-dimensional schematic representation of the cells, allowing the processes to be straightened and normalized by movement around branch points. A far greater degree of similarity is suggested from this schematic representation than is observed in their original form.

In addition to such qualitative studies, the graphic data structure permits quantification of parts of the cell which are important in determining how the intraneuronal flow of synaptic currents is achieved. Such modeling studies have been pioneered by Rall, mainly on cat spinal motor neurons (Rall, 1970). In Rall's work, many assumptions have to be made about the geometries of the dendritic processes. While such assumptions may be justified, the combination of identifiable cells and the selective staining of those cells allows the modeling of invertebrate cells with a far greater degree of precision since functional and anatomical data can be obtained from the same neuron.

The measurable parameters obtained rely on the fact that the spread of synaptic potentials depends on the "cable" properties of the neuronal processes. The equations which describe such leaky cables use the length and diameter of the process as the principal anatomical variables and the axoplasmic and membrane resistance as the main electrical ones. The most difficult values to obtain experimentally are the location of the synapses on the processes (the actual origin of the potential) and the location on the processes from which electrical measurements happen to be made.

We had hoped that double injections of functionally related cells would reveal points of contact that could reasonably be inferred to be the synaptic loci. It does appear that in some ganglia—e.g., the crayfish abdominal ganglion—the points of contact do represent synapses. However, in the lobster stomatogastric ganglion this does not appear to be the case. When points of contact seen in the fluorescent microscope were compared with electron micrographs of the same region, the apparent contacts were seen to be separated by several layers of glial sheath (D. King, unpublished observations).

Since the precise location of synapses is vital to our modeling studies, we now believe that serial electron micrographs through synaptic regions are imperative to a thorough study of these networks. Fortunately, this procedure has been aided by the discovery of several materials that not only diffuse and remain in the neuron but also contain heavy metals so that they may be seen in the electron microscope. Our procedures for reconstructing such serial electron micrographs differ from the methods used by other laboratories and will be described fully in a subsequent section.

5.1. Topological Investigation

The purpose of the schematic representation program is to compare identifiable cells in different animals topologically. An optimum representation of a cell as a two-dimensional tree is one which, in the operator's judgment, clearly brings out the placement of the largest branches, is uncluttered, and can be made to look most like the two-dimensional schematics of the same cell reconstructed from other ganglia. Figure 8 shows several such preliminary schematics. While there are gross features that tend to occur in all of them, such as the presence of a long, large secondary process near the soma with few tertiary processes emerging from it, the pictures are by no means super-imposable. Lengths, diameters, placement of branches, and number of processes vary. Similar results have been reported for other arthropod nerve cells (Cohen, 1974). The relative absence of very fine processes in some of the cells may be due to poor filling, but this is probably not the case for large secondary processes. Detailed comparisons of this sort on a large sample of suitable, well-filled, identified cells will be carried out. Since the cells exhibit the same behavior physiologically, if this study shows definite structural differences between cells, an explanation must be found. We will try to demonstrate that despite these differences the cell's functional behavior can be related to its structure. The reconstructed cells will be analyzed mathematically using

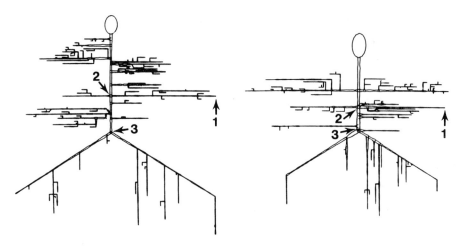

Fig. 8. Schematic representations of two PD cells from different animals, with several homologous points marked. After Selverston *et al.* (1976).

modeling techniques of the type introduced by Rall. Comparisons between them will be based on the correlation of certain network impedances and time-dependent voltage responses.

5.2. Modeling

Our model treats the reconstructed tree as many cylinders joined together. For each cylinder of length l and radius a the voltage V across the membrane, measured from the resting potential, satisfies the cable equation for passive membrane

$$\lambda^2 \frac{\partial^2 V}{\partial x^2} = V + \tau \frac{\partial V}{\partial t} \tag{1}$$

where x represents distance along the axis of the cylinder, $\lambda = [(a/2)(R_m/R_i)]^{1/2}$ is the characteristic length constant, and $\tau = R_m C_m$ is the membrane time constant. R_m is membrane resistance per unit area, and R_i is axoplasmic resistivity. This is a purely passive model, since we have not seen any experimental evidence to suggest that the processes under study have active membranes. The current I through the axoplasm along the cylinder axis obeys the equation

$$\frac{R_i}{\pi a^2} I = \frac{-dV}{dx} \tag{2}$$

Equations (1) and (2) can be solved explicitly by taking their Fourier transforms to give

$$V = A \cosh qX + B \sinh qX \qquad (3)$$

$$-\frac{R_0}{q} I = A \sinh qX + B \cosh qX \qquad (4)$$

where $q = (1 + i\omega\tau)^{1/2}$, $R_0 = R_i\lambda/\pi a^2$, $X = x/\lambda$, and A and B are constants whose values are determined by the boundary conditions.

It is most convenient to combine equations (3) and (4) into a format familiar to electrical engineers, that of coupled input–output impedance equations:

$$V_1 = R(\omega)I_1 - Q(\omega)I_2 \qquad (5)$$

$$V_2 = Q(\omega)I_1 - P(\omega)I_2 \qquad (6)$$

where V_1 and V_2 and I_1 and I_2 denote the voltage and current at $x = 0$ and $x = l$, respectively, R and P are the complex input impedances of the cylinder, and Q is the complex transfer impedance. For a passive system, these equations completely describe the response of the system if the current is specified at the points 1 and 2 as a function only of whatever lies between those two points. Expressions for R, Q, and P for a cylinder can be obtained by solving equations (3) and (4) at $x = 0$ and $x = l$, letting $L = l/\lambda$:

$$R(\omega) = P(\omega) = (R_0/q) \coth qL \qquad (7)$$

$$Q(\omega) = (R_0/q)(\sinh qL)^{-1} \qquad (8)$$

The general form represented by equations (5) and (6) completely specifies the input–output characteristics of any passive system, and the particular impedances given by equations (7) and (8) are for the case of a uniform cylinder. Obtaining the input and transfer impedances between any two points for a reconstructed cell consisting of cylinders joined together into a tree of arbitrary complexity can be done by a simple application of Kirchhoff's laws. By this means, we can obtain rules for combining such impedances in series and in parallel. For the series case (Fig. 9a), solving the equations

$$V_1 = I_1 R_A - I_2 Q_A$$
$$V_2 = I_1 Q_A - I_2 P_A = I_2 R_B - I_3 Q_B$$
$$V_3 = I_2 Q_B - I_3 P_B$$

for V_1 and V_3 in terms of I_1 and I_3 gives

$$R_{AB} = R_A - Q_A^2/(P_A + R_B)$$
$$Q_{AB} = Q_A Q_B/(P_A + R_B) \qquad \text{SERIES}$$
$$P_{AB} = P_B - Q_B^2/(P_A + R_B)$$

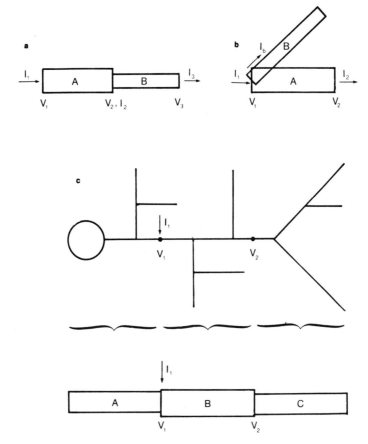

Fig. 9. Application of combination laws for cylindrical sections of membrane. (a) Two cylinders in series. (b) Two cylinders in parallel. No current flows out the end of cylinder B. (c) Reduction of a tree to three sections, the behavior of each of which is defined by its complex input and transfer impedances.

For combining two networks in parallel (Fig. 9b), we assume that the network B has no current flowing out of its terminal and hence solve the equations

$$V_1 = (I_1 - I_b)R_A - I_2 Q_A = I_b R_B$$
$$V_2 = (I_1 - I_b)Q_A - I_2 P_A$$

to give

$$\tilde{R}_{AB} = R_A R_B/(R_A + R_B)$$
$$\tilde{Q}_{AB} = Q_A R_B/(R_A + R_B) \qquad\qquad \text{PARALLEL}$$
$$\tilde{P}_{AB} = P_A - Q_A^2/(R_A + R_B)$$

The goal of this study is to use these combination rules to compare functionally identical cells according to their electrotonic properties. The following assumptions are used for the calculations:

1. The entire tree is taken to be passive, and membrane and axoplasmic resistivities are uniform everywhere. The resistivity of the extracellular medium is taken to be negligible.

2. Values for R_m and R_i are taken from the results of Hodgkin and Rushton (1946) for crab giant walking fibers but may be replaced by the results of other work in progress at our laboratory. Where available, the value of the input resistance of the entire neuron, R_N, as measured from the soma, will be compared with the computed value as a test of this.

3. All branches are treated as terminating with an infinite resistance, so that no current flows out the ends. This is because the ends are so small that their effects are negligible compared to those of the rest of the branch.

4. The soma is treated either as an isopotential object whose impedance is calculable from membrane area alone or as made up of tapered cylinders to copy the shape of the soma.

Given two reconstructed identified cells from two different animals, precisely what will we compare, and by what criteria will we compare them? Physiologically, the most meaningful quantity is the voltage as a function of time which appears at the spike-initiating zone because of integrated synaptic input. But the locations of the synapses and the spike-initiating zone, as well as the extent and strength of the synapses, are unknown. However, if we hypothesize that the spike-initiating zone lies somewhere on the process that goes out to the periphery, and a synapse might lie on branches that seem to recur from cell to cell, we may test many such pairs of points on the two cells to see how well correlated their responses are to simple inputs. Alternativley, since systems having similar impedance characteristics exhibit similar responses in the time domain, a straightforward comparison of the impedances R, Q, and P of different parts of the tree would be meaningful. Where this latter computation simply involves isolating a branch or a length of process with its attached branches from the whole structure and looking at its impedance functions, the former computation must take into account the impedance of the entire tree, not just that between the two selected points. The tree is to be reduced via the program described in Section 7.3 into three sections A, B, and C, as shown in Fig. 9c. B is part of the tree between the input and output points, A is everything before the input point, and C is the part after the output point. Then for an injected current I_1, with the assumption that no current flows out the ends of sections A and C, one can combine the input–output equations for each of the three sections. Let R_{BC} be the input impedance of the series combination of section B and section C as seen from the input point, $\tilde{R}_{A,BC}$ be the input impedance for the parallel combination of section A with the series combination of sections B and C, and $\tilde{Q}_{BC}$ be the transfer impedance of the parallel combination of sections B and C. Then one obtains

$$V_1 = I_1 \tilde{R}_{A,BC} = I_b R_{BC}$$
$$V_2 = -(-I_b)\tilde{Q}_{BC}$$

where V_1 and I_1 are the voltage and current at the input point, I_b is the current flowing through section BC at the input point, and V_2 is the voltage at the output point. This gives V_2 in terms of I_1:

$$V_2 = I_1 \tilde{Q}_{BC} R_{A,BC}/R_{BC} \tag{9}$$

and V_2 in terms of V_1:

$$V_2 = V_1 \tilde{Q}_{BC}/R_{BC} \tag{10}$$

Equations (9) and (10) relate the voltage at the output point to the voltage or current at the input point via some complex function $f(\omega)$ that can be calculated on a computer. The question remains of what basis of comparison should be used. We wish to consider both the amplitude and shape of the computed end result $f(\omega)$, since both these features are important for input–output purposes. We will use the computed value of the impedance for $\omega = 0$ (the potential reached for a step function applied current for large t) as an indication of amplitude. For comparison of shape, we will use the correlation function

$$\frac{\int_{-\infty}^{\infty} f_{c1}(\omega) f_{c2}^*(\omega) d\omega}{[\int_{-\infty}^{\infty} |f_{c1}(\omega)|^2 d\omega]^{1/2} [\int_{-\infty}^{\infty} |f_{c2}(\omega)|^2 d\omega]^{1/2}}$$

which is equal to +1 for exactly correlated functions, -1 for anticorrelated functions, and 0 for functions which are uncorrelated. The functions f_{c1} and f_{c2} will simply be the computed values of $f(\omega)$ for the two cells. This is equivalent to a comparison in the time domain of the voltage response to a delta-function current input (Section 7.4):

$$\frac{\int_0^{\infty} V_{c1}(t) V_{c2}(t) dt}{[\int_0^{\infty} V_{c1}^2(t) dt]^{1/2} [\int_0^{\infty} V_{c2}^2(t) dt]^{1/2}}$$

where the voltages are the values of V_2 from equation (9) or (10) between two 'equivalent' points on two cells being compared.

The question of dealing with synaptic input increases the difficulty of the problem, but not greatly if one uses a conductance change that is a delta function or step function in time. For any other dependence of the conductance change, the problem is much harder, although still solvable on a computer, by approximating the shape of the conductance change by a sequence of step functions or delta functions (Section 7.5).

5.3. Reconstructions from Serial Electron Micrographs

For exact, quantitative analysis of the synapse to spike-initiating zone transfer function, more precise geometric measurements are necessary than for reconstructions at the light microscopic level. Specifically, the number, distribution, total surface area, and morphology of the synaptic contacts must be determined for any realistic electrotonic cell model. It has been hypothesized (Rall and Rinzel, 1973; Barrett and Crill, 1974a,b) that synaptic morphology might be an important factor in determining "synaptic effectiveness" (the degree to which a conductance change at a synapse can effect the membrane potential at the spike initiating zone). Placement of a synapse on the tip of a small dendrite spine (as described in Purves and McMahon, 1972, for example) rather than on the surface of the dendritic cylinder itself might have a significant effect on its synaptic effectiveness. Programs have been written that enable reconstruction of synapses from serial electron micrographs, in order that their morphology may be studied more precisely. If spines or other structures which could effect synaptic effectiveness are seen to exist, the programs will be expanded to enable exact calculations of the modified electrotonic properties.

The number and distribution of synapses on a single cell can be determined only through a tedious examination of serial electron micrographs through a whole ganglion. Once reasonable values for these parameters have been determined, an estimate of total synaptic surface area could be arrived at if a value for the average synaptic surface contact area of a synapse were known. In addition to displaying the synaptic morphology, the exact area of contact between the pre- and postsynaptic processes is calculated during the reconstruction.

5.4. Procedure

Electron microscopic reconstruction studies on lobster stomatogastric ganglion neurons are just getting under way, and exact details of the procedure have not been completely worked out. It is not anticipated that our procedure will differ significantly from that used by Christensen (1973) in preparation of sea lamprey giant interneurons for electron microscopy. As was discussed above, Procion yellow is not electron opaque, and is suitable only for light microscopic studies. Christensen has found that Procion brown (MX5-BR) has all the properties desired of a stain for electron microscopy, plus many of those desired for light microscopy. Although Procion brown does not fluoresce under ultraviolet light, it does have a dark pinkish color that is readily identified in the light microscope. In addition, each molecule of the dye contains one atom of chromium, making it electron dense. Procion brown can be introduced into the cell either with pressure injection or by passing current the same as for Procion yellow, and diffuses quickly without leaking through the cell membrane.

The first steps of the procedure differ from those in Procion yellow reconstructions in the chemicals used for fixation, clearing, and embedding. Sectioning, photography, and preliminary reconstruction of the cell can be carried out as for Procion yellow fillings, although fluorescent color cues are not available. After reconstruction at the light level, any section that looks as though it might contain processes having synapses can be floated off the microscope slide, reembedded, and resectioned thin enough to be studied with an electron microscope. When a synapse is located, the serial sections through it are photographed and reconstructed as described below. The examples shown are our reconstructions from electron micrographs by Christensen of the giant axon and giant interneuron in the spinal cord of the sea lamprey *Petromyzon marinus.*

The hardware for the electron microscopic reconstructions is identical to that used for the light microscopic reconstructions. One at a time, 35-mm slides of the electron microscopic sections are rear-projected onto the data tablet, and the outlines of the portion of the processes making synaptic contact with each other are traced and stored on disk with the same program used for Procion yellow digitizations. In this case, however, the menu list is modified and assignments of indices are different:

> TYPE 1: The following points represent the outline of the presynaptic process. A "1" is entered in the index list.
> TYPE 2: The following points represent the outline of the postsynaptic process. A "2" is entered in the index list.
> TYPE 3: The following points represent the area of contact between the two process. A "3" is entered in the index list.
> TYPE 4: The following points are to be used as alignment cues, and will be deleted in the final image. A "4" is entered in the index list.
> ERASE & END: Same as for earlier program.

An example of a typical section and its digitized image is shown in Fig. 10. After all the sections through the synapse are digitized, they are aligned in exactly the same manner as are the individual films of the Procion yellow sections. For these reconstructions, no center points or diameters need be computed, so the image is thus ready for final reconstruction.

The program that constructs the final image first reads the data files

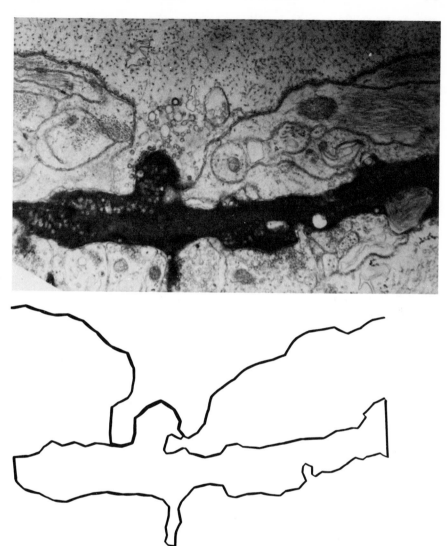

Fig. 10. Serial electron micrograph containing a process filled with Procion brown (dark area). Digitized contours of the injected cell and the presynaptic terminal are shown below.

containing the digitized section images and rearranges them into three discrete display lists, one list for each contour type discussed above (The TYPE 4 alignment cues are deleted). Next, display lists of vectors which cross-connect the contour points of adjacent sections are created. When the above lists are displayed and photographed as a stereo pair, the resultant image appears as in

Fig. 11. A calibration mark representing 1 μm is also displayed. The image can be rotated around any axis. We have found that deciphering the reconstruction is much easier when only one of the two contour types (either pre- or postsynaptic) is ribbed. This allows the observer to "look through" one end of the synapse to see the surface of the other. Another factor which greatly simplifies the image is multicolor photography. Since each contour type has its own display list, each one can be displayed individually. By making multiple exposures on the same frame of color film, each contour type being exposed through a different color filter, it is possible to obtain multicolor stereo pairs of the image from any angle.

A subroutine of the program calculates the area of the TYPE 3 contours: the surface of contact between the pre- and postsynaptic processes. This is done by dividing up the rectangles of the ribbed, fishnetlike image into triangles. The area of each triangle is calculated, and their sum is multiplied by a scaling factor computed from the calibration distance digitized on the data tablet.

6. Concluding Remarks

In this chapter we have outlined the hardware and software requirements necessary for the three-dimensional reconstruction of nerve cells. We have also indicated the types of correlated cytoarchitectural—electrophysiological studies we are undertaking using identified neurons from the lobster stomatogastric ganglion. It might be useful to speculate on what future possibilities exist for the use of computer graphics in neurobiological studies.

In terms of the analysis of small neural networks, there exists the possibility of accurately modeling the flow of subthreshold dendritic currents which result from synaptic input. Such models can eventually be incorporated into the digital network simulations, which usually consider each neuron as a point process. Repeatedly identifiable neurons also hold out the possibility of examining, in quantitative anatomical terms, the three-dimensional structure of synaptic contacts and relating it to the functional properties of that same synapse.

Anatomical studies of other invertebrate ganglia in which developmental and genetic problems are being examined will certainly be continued. Computer-aided structural studies of invertebrate neurons are only beginning but may be enormously helpful in classifying the many different types of neurons. If such reconstructions can be coupled with pattern recognition techniques, they may provide a foundation for a tractable anatomical unit analysis of the vertebrate brain.

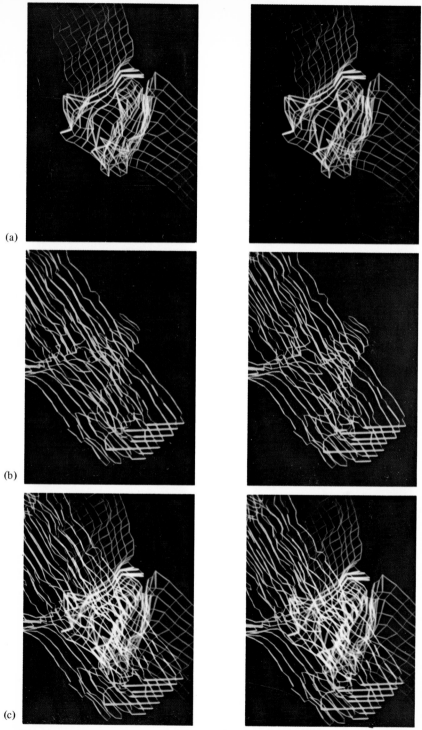

(a)

(b)

(c)

Fig. 11. Stereopairs of reconstructed synaptic terminal. (a) Presynaptic bulge. (b) Postsynaptic process. (c) Superposition of pre- and postsynaptic reconstructions.

7. Appendix

7.1. Algorithm to Draw Fat Figure

The purpose of the algorithm to draw the fat figure is to display the reconstructed tree showing the diameter information. Each segment of the tree is represented by four lines whose end-point coordinates are determined by setting up little squares around each vertex and orienting them perpendicularly to the direction of the segment. The diagonal of the square is equal to the diameter of the segment at this vertex.

Each segment is represented by a vector connecting the two vertices (vertex vector), and has two squares set up for it, one at each end. This means that each vertex also has two squares of the same size associated with it, one to be oriented perpendicular to the preceding vector, one perpendicular to the next. To build the tree display, all the vertex vectors of each segment are initially stacked along the z direction. Thus all the squares start out parallel to each other, and we can label each corner from 1 to 4 and can later join the corners with corresponding labels together. The squares surrounding the end points of each vertex vector are to be rotated about an axis perpendicular to the plane defined by the vertex vector itself and the previous vertex vector. In the case of the first vertex vector, the "previous" vector is taken in the z direction. For each pair of vertex vectors along a segment, defined by the vertex coordinates (x_1, x_2) and x_2, x_3, the steps in the computation are:

1. Compute the vectors $\mathbf{A}$ and $\mathbf{B}$ parallel to each vertex vector:

$$\mathbf{A} = x_2 - x_1 \qquad \mathbf{B} = x_3 - x_2$$

2. Compute the cosine and sine of $\mathbf{B}$ with respect to $\mathbf{A}$:

$$\cos \theta_{AB} = \mathbf{A} \cdot \mathbf{B} / |\mathbf{A}| |\mathbf{B}|$$
$$\sin \theta_{AB} = \sqrt{1 - \cos^2 \theta_{AB}}$$

3. Compute the unit vector perpendicular to $\mathbf{A}$ and $\mathbf{B}$ (axis of rotation):

$$\mathbf{C} = \mathbf{B} \times \mathbf{A} / |\mathbf{A}| |\mathbf{B}|$$

4. Compute the matrix $\mathbf{P}$ which will rotate vector $\mathbf{C}$ to the x axis, the matrix $\mathbf{M}$ which performs a rotation θ_{AB} about the x axis, and the matrix $\mathbf{P}^{-1}$ which rotates the x axis into the vector $\mathbf{C}$:

$$\mathbf{P} = \begin{vmatrix} \sin\theta\cos\phi & \sin\theta\sin\phi & \cos\theta \\ -\sin\phi & \cos\phi & 0 \\ -\cos\theta\cos\phi & -\cos\theta\sin\phi & \sin\theta \end{vmatrix}$$

$$\mathbf{M} = \begin{vmatrix} 1 & 0 & 0 \\ 0 & \cos\theta_{AB} & \sin\theta_{AB} \\ 0 & -\sin\theta_{AB} & \cos\theta_{AB} \end{vmatrix}$$

with $\cos\theta = C_z/d$, $\sin\theta = r/d$, $\sin\phi = C_x/r$, $\sin\phi = C_y/r$, $r = (C_x{}^2 + C_y{}^2)^{1/2}$, and $d = (C_x{}^2 + C_y{}^2 + C_z{}^2)^{\frac{1}{2}}$.

5. Compute $\mathbf{Q} = \mathbf{P}^{-1}\,\mathbf{MP}$, the matrix which can rotate vector **B** with respect to vector **A** about the axis **C** through an angle θ_{AB}.

6. Update cumulative rotation matrix **R** and cumulative translation vector **T**, initialized for each segment to the unit rotation matrix and zero translation vector:

$$\mathbf{R_{new}} = \mathbf{QR_{old}}$$

$$\mathbf{T_{new}} = \mathbf{QT_{old}} - \mathbf{Q}x_2 + x_2$$

7. For each point of both squares associated with the vertex vector x_2, x_3, perform the operations

$$\mathbf{x}' = \mathbf{Rx} + \mathbf{T}$$

8. After performing this operation along the entire segment, connect together the corners of the squares having the same label. Where a line associated with vertex vector x_1, x_2 intersects the next line, that associated with x_2, x_3, draw the line to the intersection point.

7.2. *Description of Algorithm to Draw Schematic*

The program to draw the schematic begins with an extremely simplistic initial configuration of the tree in two dimensions displayed graphically. The soma is represented as an ellipse. The primary process emerges from it vertically downward to its end. Secondary processes emerge horizontally from the primary process, tertiary processes emerge vertically from the secondary processes, and so on. Of the two or more segments emerging from a branch point, the one first appearing in the list, which was therefore reconstructed first, is taken to be the continuation of the branch being drawn, and the other segments emerging from the same point are defined as initial segments of higher-order branches. This representation can look very messy because of the overlapping of horizontal and vertical lines. It is the operator's task to manipulate the angles of the branches to bring out features of the schematic deemed significant. The choices he makes will take into account the diameters and lengths of the segments and features observed in schematics of the same identified cell in other animals.

To change the orientation of a branch about the point where it joins its parent branch, the operator selects the first segment of the branch with a cursor whose position is controlled by the display knobs. The display structure is then separated into two lists: one containing all the segments that can be traced to the selected segment via the FROM list, which will be manipulated as a unit and updated in software; and the rest of the tree. Each segment is characterized by three variables that determine its position and shape: a length along the segment where a bend may occur, and the angles of the pieces on either side of the bend relative to the parent segment. These three variables are manipulated on the display knobs. Software updating of the first list occurs every time an angle changes by 15° or the length changes from one vertex to the next along the segment. For each segment, the cumulative angle of its orientation is computed by tracing back via the FROM list and adding the relative angles. In this way, all parts of the branch below the segment selected for manipulation maintain the same relative orientation to it.

7.3. Description of Algorithm for Tree Computation

The algorithm which computes the complex impedances $R(\omega)$, $Q(\omega)$, and $P(\omega)$ between any two points for a tree of arbitrary complexity involves reordering the ORDER, FROM, and SEGMENT arrays (described in the text). Once the input and output points are selected, the desired ordering is one such that all segments are traceable via the FROM list to the first segment beginning at the input point and lying between the input and output points, where formerly they were traceable to the soma. This segment is redefined in the ORDER list as the first segment, and so on. In some cases, the order of a segment on the SEGMENT list will have to be reversed. After this reordering, a COUNT list is created, which contains for each segment the number of segments that lie between it and the point where it joins the line which directly connects the input and output points. Next, the impedances R, Q, and P are computed for each segment using the rule for combination in series. Then, starting with the segments having the highest value in the COUNT list, each pair of segments branching from the same parent is combined in parallel, and the result is combined in series with that parent segment and stored as that parent's impedance values. This procedure is continued down successively lower values on the COUNT list until three final sets of impedances R, Q, and P are obtained representing a network at the input end, a network lying between the input and output ends, and a network at the output end.

7.4. Correlation Function for Voltage Response

The correlation function for the voltage response at selected equivalent points on two cells has the form

$$\frac{\int_0^\infty V_{c1}(t)\,V_{c2}(t)\,dt}{\left[\int_0^\infty V_{c1}^2(t)\,dt\right]^{1/2}\left[\int_0^\infty V_{c2}^2(t)\,dt\right]^{1/2}}$$

Since $V(\omega)$, the Fourier transform of $V(t)$, is related to $I(\omega)$ by $V(\omega) = I(\omega)\,f(\omega)$, this equation can be converted to a form using impedances only, $f(\omega)$, by substituting the Fourier transform for the voltages

$$\frac{\int_0^\infty \int_{-\infty}^\infty I_{c1}(\omega)f_{c1}(\omega)e^{i\omega t}d\omega \int_{-\infty}^\infty I_{c2}(\omega')f_{c2}(\omega')e^{i\omega' t}d\omega'\,dt}{[\text{constant}]}$$

If $I_{c1}(t)$ and $I_{c2}(t)$ are delta functions in t, then $I_{c1}(\omega) = I_{c2}(\omega') = 1$, and integrating over t gives

$$\int_{-\infty}^\infty f_{c1}(\omega)\,d\omega \int_{-\infty}^\infty f_{c2}(\omega')\,d\omega' \int_0^\infty e^{i(\omega+\omega')t}\,dt$$

$$= \int_{-\infty}^\infty f_{c1}(\omega)\,d\omega \int_{-\infty}^\infty f_{c2}(\omega')\,\delta(\omega+\omega')\,d\omega'$$

$$= \int_{-\infty}^\infty f_{c1}(\omega)f_{c2}(-\omega)\,d\omega = \int_{-\infty}^\infty f_{c1}(\omega)f_{c2}^*(\omega)\,d\omega$$

Since this resultant expression has the form of a correlation function, we need only divide by the appropriate constant to obtain

$$\frac{\int_{-\infty}^\infty f_{c1}(\omega)f_{c2}^*(\omega)\,d\omega}{\left[\int_{-\infty}^\infty |f_{c1}(\omega)|^2 d\omega\right]^{1/2}\left[\int_{-\infty}^\infty |f_{c2}(\omega)|^2 d\omega\right]^{1/2}}$$

7.5. Arbitrary Synaptic Conductance Change

The cable equations for a cylinder having an excitatory conductance $G_\epsilon(T)$ across a driving potential V_ϵ, with $T = t/\tau$ and $X = x/\lambda$, are

$$\frac{\partial^2 V}{\partial X^2} = V + \frac{\partial V}{\partial T} \pm \epsilon(T)(V - V_\epsilon)$$

$$-IR_0 = \frac{\partial V}{\partial X}$$

where $\epsilon(T) = G_\epsilon R_m$. Taking the Laplace transform of the first equation in time can be done readily only for $\epsilon(T)$ having the form of a delta function or step function. For $\epsilon(T) = \epsilon_0 \delta(T)$ the equation becomes

$$\frac{d^2 V}{dX^2} = V + sV - V(0) + \epsilon_0 V(0) - \epsilon_0 V_\epsilon$$

$$= (1 + s)V - (1 - \epsilon_0) V(0) - \epsilon_0 V_\epsilon$$

While for $\epsilon(T) = \epsilon_0 u(T)$

$$\frac{d^2 V}{dX^2} = V + sV - V(0) + \epsilon_0 V - \frac{\epsilon_0 V_\epsilon}{s}$$

$$= (1 + s + \epsilon_0) V - V(X, 0) - \frac{\epsilon_0 V_\epsilon}{s}$$

These equations, incorporating an initial condition $V(0)$, have the general form

$$\frac{d^2 V}{dX^2} = p^2 V - f(X, 0) - g(s)$$

The solution for this equation is

$$V = A \cosh pX + B \sinh pX + \frac{g(s)}{p^2} - \tfrac{1}{2}e^{pX} \int e^{-2pX} dX \int e^{pX} f(X) \, dX$$

$$- \tfrac{1}{2}e^{-pX} \int e^{2pX} dX \int e^{-pX} f(X) \, dX$$

Thus equations for voltage and current have the form

$$V = A \cosh pX + B \sinh pX + F(s) - G(X, s)$$

$$\frac{-IR_0}{p} = A \sinh pX + B \cosh pX - \frac{dG}{dX}$$

Evaluating these equations at $X = 0$ and $X = L$ gives coupled input–output equations

$$V_1 = I_1 R - I_2 Q + F(s) + \frac{1}{\sinh pL} \frac{dG}{dx} \bigg|_L$$

$$V_2 = I_1 Q - I_2 P + F(s) - G + \coth pL \frac{dG}{dx} \bigg|_L$$

where R, Q, and P have the same form as appears in the text for a cylinder. These equations can be used to obtain expanded rules for combination of cylinders. Thus an arbitrarily shaped conductance can be solved using this method by approximating it as a sequence of step functions or delta functions.

8. References

Barrett, J. N., and Crill, W. E., 1974*a*, Specific membrane properties of cat motoneurones, *J. Physiol. (London)* **239**:301–324.

Barrett, J. N., and Crill, W. E., 1974*b*, Influence of dendritic location and membrane properties on the effectiveness of synapses on cat motoneurones, *J. Physiol. (London)* **239**:325–345.

Christensen, B., 1973, Procion brown: An intracellular dye for light and electron microscopy, *Science* **182**:1255–1256.

Cohen, M. J., 1974, Trophic interactions in excitable systems of invertebrates, *Ann. N.Y. Acad. Sci.* **228**:364–380.

Hodgkin, A. L., and Rushton, W. A. H., 1946, The electrical constants of a crustacean nerve fibre, *Proc. R. Soc. London Ser. B* **133**:444–449.

Purves, D., and McMahon, W., 1972, The distribution of synapses on a physiologically identified motor neuron in the CNS of the leech, *J. Cell Biol.* **55**:205–220.

Rall, W., 1970, Cable properties of dendrites and effect of synaptic location, in: *Excitatory Synaptic Mechanisms*, (P. Anderson and J. K. S. Jansen, eds.), UniversitetsforLaget, Oslo.

Rall, W., and Rinzel, J., 1973, Branch input resistance and steady state attenuation for input to one branch of a dendritic neuron model, *Biophys. J.* **13**:648.

Selverston, A. I., 1973, The use of intracellular dye injections in the study of small neural networks, in: *Intracellular Staining in Neurobiology* (S. B. Kater and C. Nicholson, eds.), pp. 255–280, Springer–Verlag, New York.

Selverston, I., Russell, D. F., Miller, J. P., and King, D. G., 1976, The stomatogastric nervous system: Structure and function of a small neural network, *Prog. Neurobiol.* (in press).

Wann, D., Woolsley, T., Dierker, R., and Cowan, M., 1973, An on-line digital computer system for the semiautomatic analysis of Golgi-impregnated neurons, *IEEE Trans. Biomed. Eng.* **20**:233–247.

Ware, R., 1972 Thesis, Columbia University.

3

A Measuring System for Analyzing Neuronal Fiber Structure

A. Paldino and E. Harth

1. Introduction

Structure and function are the two properties of any biological system that challenge our understanding. But nowhere is structure more complex or function more obscure than in the mammalian central nervous system. Certainly, any progress in our understanding of cerebral function requires us to know more about brain structure. But the converse is also true. Since a precise specification of the vast neural network encountered, for example, in the cerebal cortex is out of the question, we must ask what are the functionally significant parameters of neural structure. Thus the prejudices of the experimenter are unfortunately imprinted on the investigations at the outset, and we should be aware of some inevitable circularity in our approach.

The cytoarchitectonics of neural tissue has been studied by many methods and on different scales, from the gross features apparent to the naked eye to details of individual synapses visible only under the electron microscope. In the intermediate range of optical microscopy, we are aided by a great variety of staining techniques which have been employed to emphasize particular features. The different types of Golgi stains are characterized by high-contrast staining of individual neurons, including their entire dendritic tree and sometimes the entire axon with all of its ramifications. This method was used extensively in the classification of cell types and their distribution in the nervous system, but its use in determining properties of the neural network was limited by a few shortcomings: The stains selected a relatively small fraction of all neurons for

A. Paldino · Department of Neuroscience, Rose Fitzgerald Kennedy Center for Research in Mental Retardation and Human Development, Albert Einstein College of Medicine, Bronx, New York 10461. *E. Harth* · Physics Department, Syracuse University, Syracuse, New York 13210.

complete staining, leaving all others invisible. The physical basis of the selectivity is unknown. Thus functional connections between neurons were observed relatively rarely in Golgi stains, and never with absolute certainty. Quantitative data were cumbersome to extract, depending for the most part on elaborate camera lucida drawings of the microscope image. Furthermore, such measurements were almost entirely confined to cell parts visible in one tissue section (typically about 100 μm thick), since no method existed for efficient coordinate transformation from one section to the next.

In the present work, we are trying to overcome some of these difficulties, and thus render the Golgi method a more efficient tool of research. Underlying the work will be the assumption that important information concerning neural connectivity can be derived without observation of the synapses by a statistical investigation of dendritic and axonal fiber densities as functions of location in the cortex and location of the parent cell. This requires first the ability to follow structures from one microsection to another. For rough alignment, natural or artificial fiducial features can be used. The rhinal fissures or one of the cerebral ventricles can be used for this purpose, as well as notches cut into the tissue. For the precise coordinate transformation required at high magnification, local features (e.g., exiting fibers) must be used. For this purpose, we have developed a procedure in which a set of exiting fiber points is measured on the two adjacent surfaces of a given pair of sections. A computer program, called *MATCH*, will then find the appropriate transformation parameters. This is described in Section 3.3.

The method presupposes a high degree of dimensional stability of the tissue. We have found that the traditional method of paraffin embedding is unsuitable for this purpose but that celloidin (manufactured by E. I. du Pont de Nemours Co. under the trade name Parlodion) possesses both required stability and ease of slicing. We have used entire rat brains embedded in celloidin after fixing and staining. Serial sections (80–100 μm thick) are readily prepared and mounted on microslides for analysis.

The aim in the current study is to obtain parameters describing the structure of neocortex on a scale of the order of the size of the functional columns reported in both the visual and somatosensory cortex (Hubel and Wiesel, 1962, 1963, 1968, Mountcastle, 1957). Hence typical analysis involves regions of the order of millimeters. Measurements are taken on rapid Golgi, Golgi–Cox, and Nissl stains of the same cortical regions.

Measurements on cells and fibers are carried out by a video digitizer described in Section 2. The microscope image is displayed on a TV screen and point measurements are taken by a cursor spot which is under manual control. A rotary encoder attached to the fine-focusing control of the microscope provides the third coordinate. The system is linked via a teletype terminal and telephone coupler to the PDP-10 computer of the Syracuse University Computing Center. Some of the programs used in analysis of the data are described in Section 3.

2 Instrumentation: The Video Digitizer

2.1. Optical System

A Leitz Ortholux research microscope is used, equipped with gauge micrometers to read (to 2 μm) translations of the stage along two Cartesian axes. We use plano objective lenses (4x, 10x, 25x, 40x) and a 100:1 oil immersion objective. Plano eyepieces (10x, 25x) are used to increase the flatness of the image field. The image is picked up by a GE 875 closed-circuit TV camera, and displayed on a 23-inch television screen (Conrac CVA23 with GE4TE21A1BA monitor interface). Lower magnifications are used primarily for orienting purposes. Most measurements are taken at 250x magnification, while oil immersion is used occasionally when high resolution is required. The diaphragm in the condenser stage of the microscope is fully opened to provide the smallest possible depth of focus. When operated in this way, depth discrimination by means of the fine-focusing adjustment is reproducible to within about 1 μm.

2.2. Control Digitizer

The control digitizer, constructed from integrated circuits, performs the following functions:

1. It generates on the TV face a cursor spot whose position is manually controlled by a *MOUSE* (a device, manufactured by Adage, Inc., Frazer/Malvern, Pa, mounted on two wheels, perpendicular to one another, which are shaft-mounted to two single-turn potentiometers).
2. It converts the cursor coordinates, X_c, Y_c, to digital information and visually displays its position as three-digit numbers.
3. It converts the output of a rotary encoder, Z_c, to digital information and displays this as a third three-digit number.
4. It transmits the X_c, Y_c, Z_c coordinate information of cursor and fine focusing along with a code number (0–15) indicating the nature of a particular point that has been measured (e.g., branch point, cell body location, fiber start, fiber end) to a PDP-10 computer via a teletype terminal and telephone coupler.

To achieve these functions, the digitizer is composed of four subsystems, shown schematically in Fig. 1. These are the visual display, axis difinition, point generation, and teletype output. The description, construction, details, and interconnections of these four subsystems are given below.

The *visual display subsystem* converts manual input positional information to TTL (transistor–transistor logic) compatible logic levels defining nine digits

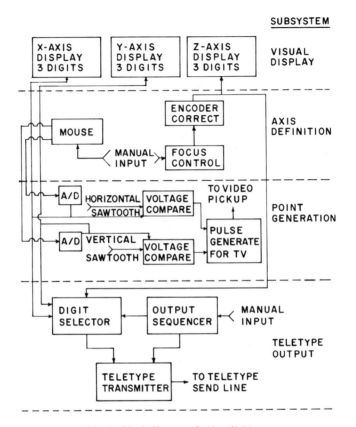

Fig. 1. Block diagram of video digitizer.

of BCD (binary-coded decimal) information. Three Sperry SP-753 (Sperry Information Displays Division, Scottsdale, Ariz.) information displays are used. These devices are of bar construction whose character size is 0.27 by 0.55 inch. A minimum recommended voltage of 170 V DC is required to ionize the display. A DD-700 decoder/driver (a monolithic integrated circuit providing the seven-segment SP-753 information displays) is required for each digit. Codes representing the numbers 10–15 are decoded to display the letters A–F.

Axis definition is derived by the MOUSE. It is used here to locate a cursor on the screen of the TV monitor. The MOUSE rests on two wheels perpendicular to each other whose shafts are mounted on low-torque potentiometers. Movement of the MOUSE causes its wheels to resolve the motion into its X and Y components. The potentiometers convert the X,Y travel into analog voltages which are then externally processed by two analog-to-digital (A/D) converters. The output of the A/D converters is used as input to the X,Y visual display. The

A/D converters used are Datel model ADC-K12B (Datel Systems, Inc., Canton, Mass., formerly Varadyne Systems). These have an output resolution of 12 binary digits. The X, Y visual display is in hexadecimal notation. It is converted into decimal notation by subroutine IN.MAC (a subprogram of MAMS.F4 described in Section 3) which receives hexadecimal input and outputs this in decimal notation.

The Z-coordinate corresponds to the depth in the tissue section. It is obtained from a rotary-shaft encoder mounted on the fine-focusing knob of the microscope. The 1000 counts/rev Datex (Datex Corp., Monrovia, Calif.) encoder measures angular shaft position by the use of coded disks and associated brushes. The coded disks are divided into a number of positions, each discrete position being defined by a unique combination of contact closures. The contact arrangement is formed by a number of brushes contacting a photoetched pattern on the disk. The output from the encoder must be processed by an encoder-correct logic board which converts this output into BCD to be used as input to the Z-axis visual display coordinate.

The *point generation subsystem* injects a spot into a video signal at the two-dimensional point defined by six of the BCD digits provided by the axis definition subsystem. This is accomplished by using the unconverted analog voltage from the MOUSE (X, Y coordinates) and the TV monitor sawtooth voltage as inputs to a voltage comparator. The outputs from the two voltage comparators are processed by two TTL monostable (Fairchild 9600DC) retriggerable resettable monostable multivibrators, the outputs of which are then AND-gated, inverted, and relayed to the video pickup. In Fig. 2, C_x, C_y and

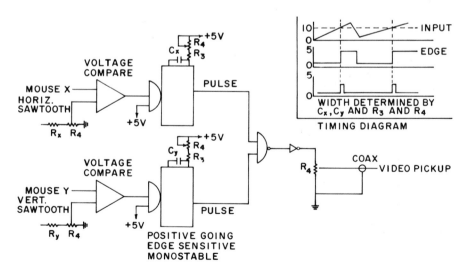

Fig. 2. Pulse generation scheme.

R_x, R_y have different values to adjust the different sawtooth voltages available and axis time windows desired. The sawtooth R_4 control must be internal as it defines the relation between video picture position and digital numbers, but the R_4 which is coupled to C_x and C_y is remote for manual adjustment of point size. The R_4 variable resistance off the coax varies the point brightness $(R_4 = 0–10 \text{ k}\Omega, C_{x,y} = 100 \text{ pf}, R_3 = 5 \text{ k}\Omega)$. The voltage comparators used are Fairchild linear I.C. U9A7734393.

The *teletype output subsystem* generates and transmits ASCII teletype code for each of the nine digits provided by the axis definition subsystem. Coupled with the digit selector, a coordinate and its associated code are transmitted (refer to Fig. 3 for the logic of the digit selector.)

In general, the transmission is in the following sequence:

$$C \qquad XXX \qquad YYY \qquad ZZZ$$

where C is a number from 0 to 15 corresponding to the code of that particular point. X, Y represent a digit from 0 to 9 or a letter from A to F, and Z is a digit from 0 to 9. The X, Y, Z binary characters are processed mainly by the subsystem which accepts binary characters from a terminal device and receives/transmits these characters with appended control and error-detecting bits. The device used is a UAR/T universal asynchronous receiver/transmitter model AY-5-1012 from GIANT (General Instrument Advanced Nitride Tech-

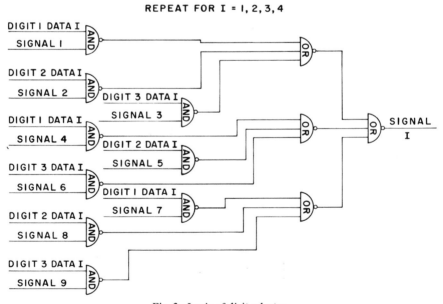

Fig. 3. Logic of digit selector.

nology, Inc., via Summit Distributors, Buffalo, N.Y.). This is a 40-lead dual inline package.

The code is processed by a Fairchild 9318DC eight-input priority encoder designed to accept eight inputs and produce a binary weighted code of the highest-order input. The number of codes is doubled to 16 by inserting a two-position switch between +5 V and ground on the most significant bit of a Fairchild 9312DC eight-input multiplexer.

The transmission of the code and coordinate is sent over teletype cable to a telephone coupler (Omnitec Corp, Phoenix, Ariz., model 701A) which interfaces the teletype with the PDP-10 computer. Table I is a parts list for each subsystem, and Fig. 1 is a block diagram of the video digitizer.

Table I. Parts List

Subsystem	Part	Number required
Visual display	Sperry SP-753	3
	DD-700 decoder/driver	9
Axis definition	Fairchild 9016DC	3
	Fairchild 9017DC	1
	Fairchild 9002DC	3
	Fairchild 9014DC	3
Point generation	ADC-K12B (A/D)	2
	UA734	2
	Fairchild 9600DC	2
	Fairchild 9016DC	1
	Fairchild 9002DC	1
Teletype output	Fairchild 9312DC	4
	Fairchild 9322DC	2
	Fairchild 9000DC	1
	Fairchild 9602DC	1
	Fairchild 9310DC	1
	Fairchild 9017DC	1
	Fairchild 9318DC	1
	UAR/T GI7314	1

The power requirements are met with the following power supplies:

Input	Power required	Part
115 VAC	+5 VDC, 3.0 A	Power/mate EM-5B
115 VAC	±12 VDC, 1.5 A	Power/mate EM-12B
115 VAC	±15 VDC, 30 mA	Datel BPM-15/30
+5 VDC	200 VDC (two required)	Sperry VC-523

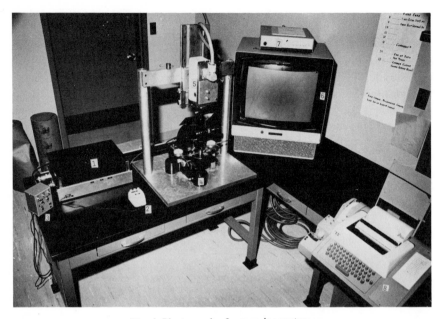

Fig. 4. Photograph of measuring system.

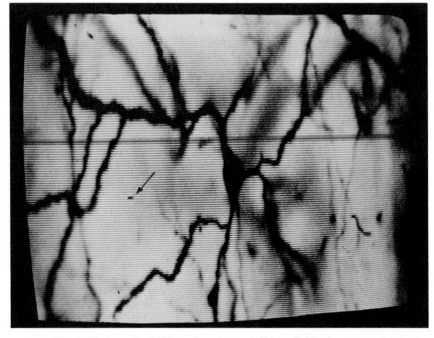

Fig. 5. Photograph of TV monitor. Arrow indicates digitized cursor spot.

Appropriate capacitor values are wired into all subsystems to reduce noise due to effects of line voltage variations and TV monitor operation and to reduce the flickering rate of the visual displays.

Figure 4 shows the measuring system. Included in this photograph are the control digitizer (1), MOUSE (2), code (function) box (3), microscope (4), closed-circuit TV camera (5), TV monitor (6), camera—monitor interface (7), and teletype (8). Figure 5 shows the TV monitor with an image of a rapid Golgi stained neuron. The arrow locates the digitized cursor spot.

3. Software

3.1. Standardization of Video Screen

When a data point is first recorded, the coordinates of the cursor spot must be transformed such that they are anchored in a coordinate system common to all points. The digital information of the coordinates of the cursor is displayed as a three-digit number in hexadecimal notation. This is the result of using two A/D converters which have an output resolution of 12 binary bits. The advantage of using these converters is that the count range of the cursor spot is increased from 0–999 (decimal notation) to 0–4069 in both X and Y count coordinates.

To convert cursor coordinates from counts to distances (in micrometers), we must calibrate the surface of the TV. This was accomplished by placing a micrometer slide with divisions of 10 μm on the microscope stage and obtaining cursor count coordinates over a matrix of known positions over the entire field. In this way, it was found that the relationship between cursor counts and distances in micrometers could be approximated to a high degree of accuracy, for both the X and Y coordinates, by a quadratic of the form

$$d_x = \alpha_x (\xi - \xi_0) + \beta_x (\xi - \xi_0)^2$$

and a similar expression for d_y. Here d_x, d_y are the Cartesian coordinates (in micrometers) from the upper right corner of the screen, ξ, η are cursor coordinates (in counts), ξ_0, η_0 are cursor coordinates (in counts) at the upper right corner of the screen, α_x, α_y are linear magnifications (micrometers/counts), and β_x, β_y are second-order correction terms (micrometers/counts^2). We found that for our system the second-order correction terms β_x and β_y are small but not insignificant.

Finally, a transformation is carried out into a coordinate system fixed in the tissue rather than on the TV screen, thus allowing for motions of the microscope stage. For this purpose, the micrometer gauge settings Ξ, H are combined with the TV coordinates d_x, d_y to give coordinates in the tissue section being measured:

$$X = \Xi + \alpha_x^{(i)} \left[(\xi - \xi_0) + \frac{\beta_x^{(i)}}{\alpha_x^{(i)}} (\xi - \xi_0)^2 \right] + \Delta X^{(i)}$$

$$Y = H + \alpha_y^{(i)} \left[(\eta - \eta_0) + \frac{\beta_y^{(i)}}{\alpha_y^{(i)}} (\eta - \eta_0)^2 \right] + \Delta Y^{(i)}$$

where $\alpha_x^{(i)}, \alpha_y^{(i)}$ refer to the magnifications defined previously for a particular objective lens. The change of objective lenses by rotation of the microscope turret also involves a parallel displacement of the lens axis. This is taken into account by the terms $\Delta X^{(i)}, \Delta Y^{(i)}$, which measure displacements relative to the axis of the 25x objective lens. Thus measurements can be carried out at the magnification convenient to the operator.

Repeated measurements of at least two identifiable points make the determination of the coefficients a straightforward task.

The Z coordinate is easily computed. One revolution of the fine-focus control moves the microscope stage through a true distance of 157.4 μm. This corresponds to a count difference from the rotary encoder of 1000 counts. Therefore, the Z coordinate is transformed as follows:

$$Z = Z_c/6.36 \pm 1 \ \mu m$$

where Z_c is the count reading from rotary encoder (decimal notation) and Z is the coordinate (micrometers). As noted previously, the Z coordinate represents the depth into the tissue of the data point.

3.2. MAMS.F4 (MOUSE-Assisted Measuring System) Program

The micrometer gauge settings of the microscope stage are not digitized automatically because of the relative infrequency of their adjustment. The readings are taken by the operator and communicated to the computer via the teletype along with specifications of the objective lens and a code describing the type of data point measured. The X, Y, Z coordinates are sent to the computer whenever a measuring button is pressed. After carrying out the coordinate transformations described above, the computer stores on disk, for every point measured, the following information:

1. Slide set (this is to identify the series to which histological data point belongs).
2. Slide number.
3. Cell number.
4. Fiber number.

5. Point number.
6. Code.
7. *X*, *Y*, and *Z*.

The program, of course, has various checks written into it. Examples are:

1. It compares the slide set and slide number under consideration with the data already on the disk to inform the operator if data had been previously recorded from this pair.
2. It determines if the data point is within a specified distance (usually 5–10 μm) of any other data point already recorded from the same slide set and slide number and, if so, informs the operator of the actual distance from this point and gives the operator the option of recording the current data point in memory.
3. It allows the operator to erase the previously measured data point from core.
4. It allows for comments to change
   a. Slide set.
   b. Slide number.
   c. Scale (magnification).
   d. Cell number.
   e. Fiber number.
   f. Point number.
   g. Micrometer setting of microscope.

The accumulated data are recorded on DECtapes.

3.3. MATCH.F4 Program

The purpose of MATCH.F4 is to determine the section-to-section transformation coefficients between serial sections that enable us to locate rapidly a fiber continuing from one section to another. The program reads the data recorded on disk by the MAMS program and enters into an array only data points having the code 8 or 9 from the same slide set and two consecutive slide numbers. Code 8 indicates a point at which a fiber has been determined to exit or enter the lower surface of slide k, and code 9 indicates a point at which a fiber exits or enters the upper surface of slide $k + 1$. Of course, great care has been taken to ensure that exiting and entering points are roughly in the same area under consideration in both slides. Natural features and/or fiducial marks placed in the tissue prior to sectioning will facilitate this procedure. To obtain the translation and rotation parameters that give precise alignment, the following algorithms is applied: the distances between all pairs of points are calculated for both surfaces. Let $r_{i,j}(k)_L$ be the distance between points i and j on the lower surface of slide k. Similarly, let $r_{m,n}(k+1)_u$ be the distance between points m and n on the upper surface of slide $k+1$. The distance $r_{1,2}(k)_L$ is compared with all $r_{m,n}(k+1)_u$ until a distance match (usually within a 5 μm tolerance) is found. If no distance match is noted, $r_{1,3}(k)_L$ is then compared with all $r_{m,n}(k+1)_u$. When a distance match is found, the orientations of these distances are then compared and represent a tentative match if the angle between the two is $10°$ or less. (One knows *a priori* that the tissue slices are mounted on the slide such that the angular orientation is much less than $10°$.) Suppose the distance $r_{4,7}(k)_L$ matches the distance $r_{8,13}(k+1)_u$ and their orientations are also within the tolerance range.

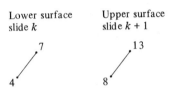

All distances $r_{4,j}(k)_L$ $(j \neq 4,7)$ are then compared with all $r_{8,l}(k+1)_u$ $(l \neq 8,13)$.

Let us suppose that points 14 and 3 satisfy both orientation and distance criteria:

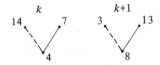

If now $r_{7,14}(k)_L$ matches $r_{3,13}(k+1)_u$ then the points 4, 7, and 14 in k are said to form a triplet match with 8, 13, and 3 in section $k+1$. A least-squares fit is then performed on these points such that the resultant transformation coefficients minimize the sum of the squares of the distances between corresponding points.

When a triplet match is found, the program searches for a fourth point. The final transformation coefficients are determined by considering all sets of triplet and quadruplet matches.

4. Conclusion

The video digitizer is suitable for a variety of anatomical investigations. Utilizing Nissl-stained nervous tissue, one may accurately and easily perform cell density measurements. With the two common modifications of the Golgi technique (Golgi–Cox and rapid Golgi), one is able to record the neuronal network of neurons. Significant studies which can be performed on these data include (1) polar and azimuth angle distributions of axon and dendritic collaterals, (2) branching angles of fibers, (3) distribution of fiber end points terminating within the tissue volume, (4) spine distributions, (5) cell-type distributions, and (6) integrated fiber-length distributions.

Program NERVE, which utilizes the PDP-10-VB10C graphics terminal at Syracuse University, reconstructs the three-dimensional data on disk and displays the fiber image. From the terminal, the operator is able to translate and rotate the image with respect to any of the three axes. This method employing *real-time* control over the orientation of the projection plane is particularly useful in looking for asymmetries in the fiber network.

ACKNOWLEDGMENTS

The authors wish to acknowledge technical assistance by Mr. C. McCarthy in connection with the design of the video digitizer. This research was supported in part by grant NS 10917 from the National Institutes of Health.

5. References

Hubel, D. H., and Wiesel, T. N., 1962, Receptive fields, binocular interaction and functional architecture in the cat's visual cortex, *J. Physiol. (London)* **160**:106–154.
Hubel, D. H., and Wiesel, T. N., 1963, Shape and arrangement of columns in cat's striate cortex, *J. Physiol. (London)* **165**:559–570.
Hubel, D. H., and Wiesel, T. N., 1968, Receptive fields and functional architecture of monkey striate cortex, *J. Physiol. (London)* **195**:215–243.
Mountcastle, V. B., 1957, Modality and topography properties of single neurons of cat's somatic sensory cortex, *J. Neurophysiol.* **20**:408–434.

4

Automatic and Semiautomatic Analysis of Nervous System Structure

D. E. Hillman, R. Llinás, and M. Chujo

1. Introduction

Interdisciplinary approaches to the study of neuronal structure and function have provided the opportunity to develop an automatic and reliable method for three-dimensional reconstruction, analysis, and storage of morphological data. Today, varied types of images, at light microscopic and ultrastructural levels, are obtained from morphological as well as physiological (Kater and Nicholson, 1973) and cytochemical techniques (Smith *et al.*, 1974). Their levels of magnification range from macroscopic projections of brain surfaces in serial sections to ultramicroscopic detail of intracellular particles and organelles. Thus a system capable of automatically processing such information is of central importance if morphological studies are to be based on more than casual observation. The system should have the capability of semiautomated and manual input control for the processing of difficult material.

Two basic approaches have proven possible for this purpose. *Perimeter extraction* has been utilized for many years as a means of reconstructing surfaces of internal CNS structures in three dimensions (Born, 1883; Conradi, 1969). From sectioned material, cell surfaces were assembled utilizing stacked sheets of wax, plastic, cardboard, or other materials. Levinthal and Ware (1972) and Willey *et al.* (1973) have extended this technique to computerized recording from outlines of profiles obtained on structures in serial sections. Profile stacking has allowed this approach to define the course of complex fibers in the neuropil; it has also been used to define cell-surface configurations (Levinthal *et al.*, 1974).

D. E. Hillman, R. Llinás, and M. Chujo • Department of Physiology and Biophysics, New York University Medical Center, 550 First Avenue, New York, New York 10016.

The second approach utilizes sequential reconstruction of cell processes by defining their patterns of tridimensional distribution as axial coordinates. This we call the *vector-branching mode*. Morphologists have used a similar two-dimensional approach for portraying cells since Golgi (1873) discovered his famous "black reaction" as a means of visualizing neural elements. Computer-aided reconstruction was first utilized by Glaser and Van der Loos (1965). With more advanced technology, others have extended this application (Coleman *et al.*, 1973; Hillman *et al.*, 1974; Lindsay and Scheibel, 1974; Llinás and Hillman, 1975; Reddy *et al.*, 1973; Selverston, 1973; Wann *et al.*, 1973). Basically this approach has two versions. In one, the cell processes are recorded as they are followed through thick sections. The *Z* coordinate is obtained by carefully determining the depth of the structure within sections, taking advantage of the short focal depth of high-magnification microscope lenses (optical sectioning). The reconstruction of cell processes starts at an arbitrary point, usually the soma, and vectors or closely aligned points are used to reconstruct the tridimensional distributions of the processes. At bifurcation points, each successive branch segment is followed to include its branches and ultimately its terminals. This is designated as *vector-branching–optical-sectioning mode* (VB-OSM).

The other version of this approach has been developed to accommodate reconstruction from serially sectioned material (Llinás and Hillman, 1975; Reddy *et al.*, 1973; Selverston, 1973). It requires a more elaborate method; thus the sections must be accurately aligned such that components of each section share a strict match. After recording the coordinates for the processes within individual sections and assembling them in "pages" in computer memory, the software which assembles the tree must be capable of organizing the data as consecutive points beginning at a point of origin and arranging them in the proper space dimensions. The algorithm involves matching closest points between the aligned pages. This approach is designated *vector-branching–page mode* (VB-PM).

Our tridimensional neuronal reconstruction system utilizes the PDP-15 graphics display implementation, which allows rotation and the utilization of online interactive subroutines, all of which are particularly valuable in the analysis of form. Besides giving an accurate conceptual image of the neuronal form under study, it provides important clues for the design of new morphological and physiological studies. The analysis, which can be quantitative, is essential for the evaluation of comparative features between cells of a given class, as well as within different cell classes. The analysis of suitable numbers of cells allows the acquisition of information regarding the stochastic and invariant aspects of an idealized neuronal form (Hillman *et al.*, 1974; Lindsay and Scheibel, 1974; Llinás and Hillman, 1975). The analytical power of such a system is of interest, especially with regard to study of the functional properties of individual neurons as well as entire groups of cells.

2. Multipurpose Three-Dimensional Recording System

2.1. General Aspects

The system described here has the capability of recording either "axial coordinates" of neuronal trees or "perimeters" for surface contours. Perimeter-recorded data can also be used for extraction of the axial coordinates. This system enables automated, semiautomated, and manually implemented input procedures to be utilized with the same hardware. When the complexity of the structures exceeds the image-recognition capability of a given system, automated methods fail. In these cases, the cells must be recorded with interactive aids.

Given the wealth of detail and the quantity of information available on nervous system structure, data reduction is an important requirement even with present computer capabilities. The methodology utilized for such data reduction varies with the approaches of different laboratories. The actual implementation of data-reduction routines is largely governed by the form of the material and the hardware available. Since light and electron optical images are the principal source of material for study, certain restrictions are placed on thickness of specimens to be reconstructed. In preparations from invertebrates which contain cells injected with intracellular dyes (Murphey, 1973; Pitman *et al.*, 1973), very thick preparations may be used. On the other hand, in cases where the material is stained by perfusion or immersion techniques, such as the Golgi method, the sections are usually limited to about 150 μm because of residual staining components in the tissue or density of the impregnated elements. When small or numerous overlapping structures are present within a specific region, such as often happens in light microscopic sections, thin serial sections are required. Likewise, fluorescent dye injected cells of the vertebrate CNS must be sectioned for clear definition of their processes because of background fluorescence due to fixation (Kater *et al.*, 1973). At the ultrastructural level, ultra-thin sections must be used in order to define membrane structures and synaptic relationships.

These varied conditions require a multipurpose application of hardware. In cases where thick preparations allow "optical sectioning" of the entire structure in one slide, the solution is simple. When thin-sectioned material is to be used, structures must be extracted from component pages. Since most neurons extend beyond the thickness of the usual Golgi section (100 μm), a combination of optical sectioning and reconstruction from pages is necessary in order to capture the entire extent of the dendritic processes. Likewise, the higher magnifications needed to resolve fine branching and discrete processes demand that sequentially obtained information be compiled from numerous fields in order to reconstruct the entire structure. These constraints require rather complex software programs and necessitate the use of varied hardware applications.

Our own approach to this problem is based on hardware data reduction, utilizing automated perimeter extraction or interactive input of perimeters and axial coordinates for tree structures. A discussion of our hardware and interfacing configuration for tridimensional reconstruction and other general applications of this technique to neurobiology is given in Llinás and Hillman (1975).

2.2. Description of the System

2.2.1. Computer Hardware

Basically our system consists of a PDP-15 computer with 28 K memory (18 bits/word) and graphics capability interfaced to a Quantimet 720 image analysis system (Fig. 1). Peripherals essential to the recording procedure are a writing tablet with coordinate processor, A/D converter, fixed-head disk, display processor and graphics display, paper tape punch, and relay drivers. The interfacing consists of (1) a writing tablet coordinate processor to the variable frame and scale of the Quantimet 720, and (2) an interface of the X, Y coordinate system of the Quantimet to a memory buffer, which in turn is interfaced to software-controlled relay drivers which activate stepping motors to control the microscope stage in the X and Y directions. A stepping motor on the focus control of the microscope changes the Z coordinate and is sensed by potentiometer feedback to the A/D converter in the optical-sectioning mode.

2.2.2. Software and Input Procedure

Two basic routines being applied in our research include either perimeter extraction or the vector-branching recording for three-dimensional reconstruction. A number of subroutines have been developed in order to accommodate the various input configurations. Each program may be used with all options. Since these options require large amounts of core memory, some may be deleted in order to allow recording of a larger number of data points. The size of effective programs has been found to be in the range of 20 K words. A core memory of 32 or 64 K words is very advantageous with the present configuration.

2.2.2a. Perimeter Extraction. Two basic approaches to perimeter extraction are being used: (1) manual input and (2) automated input. In the former case, the spark pen is employed in an *interactive mode* to follow outlines of desired structures while recording the X, Y coordinates. The number of X, Y points necessary to describe a complex perimeter is reduced by eliminating those details which fall close to a linear excursion. Thus the number of points needed to specify a perimeter is directly proportional to the level of detail sought.

The traced images may be taken from photographs, from drawings, or

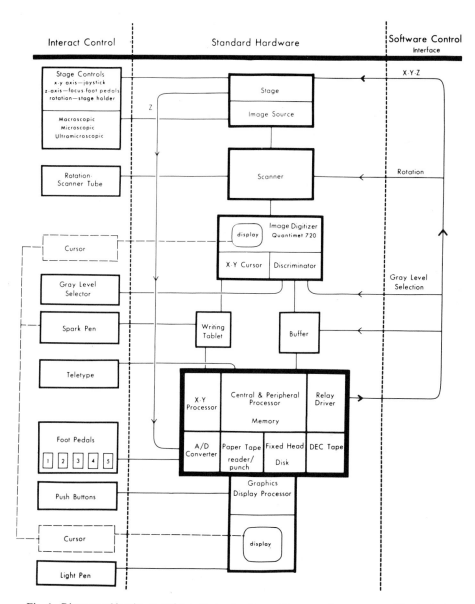

Fig. 1. Diagram of hardware and interfacing for the multipurpose input system. Histological information is recorded automatically or interactively by the same system. In addition, branching-tree structures can be reconstructed through optical sectioning or through actual serial sections.

directly from the preparation through the image-analyzing computer (IAC). In the latter case, the writing-tablet-controlled cursor system on the PDP-15 graphics computer is interfaced to allow spark-pen control of a cursor on the IAC display. The cursor on the image display is used to follow the outline and thus the writing tablet processor serves to specify simultaneously the coordinates for recording the perimeters. Multiple perimeters can be recorded as different objects or parts of the same form.

The operation is relatively simple since structures are easily traced and instructions to the computer are at the operator's direct command. For example after tracing each perimeter, completion is signaled by a push button on the graphic display, which activates the closure of the perimeter by automatically connecting the last and first points recorded. Other perimeters can be recorded on the same page level and similarly closed. A new page recording is initiated by a second push button. The traced outline of the previous page remains on the screen, at a lower intensity, for reference. Perimeters are stored to be used in the rotation program described below (see Fig. 2).

The *automated perimeter extraction* (APE) method utilizes the surface contour extracted directly from thin or thick sections via the IAC. In this case, gray-level detection is used to select data from stained or reacted material. The area or perimeter of desired objects on a section or at a focal plane is selected by windowing the gray level on the IAC display system (Fig. 3 top). The coordinates for these picture points are then transferred to a buffer memory system (BMS) which serves as an interface between the two computers. The PDP-15 software is designed so that data points can be read from the BMS and perimeter points for vectors which outline the object are produced by a search for the perimeter of each object. The outlines are projected onto the graphics display (Fig. 3 bottom). At this point, the operator can choose to interact with the recorded data in order to DELETE (Fig. 3) or amend the data if necessary. This is carried out by an interactive light pen on the graphics screen.

The entire recording is automated by software control of the focal drive and BMS (Fig. 1) which allows optical sectioning. If there are a number of sections on the same slide, successive sections are aligned using the previous recorded image. Only those objects which are of a spherical nature are used for the alignment procedure, thus minimizing drifts. This procedure is carried out utilizing the stage X and Y control and rotation on the scanner in order to achieve best fit for selected objects. This eliminates the photographic superimposition of images as an intermediate step described by Levinthal and Ware (1972).

In the APE procedure, the basic data reduction is made first at the specimen level by selective staining and later at the computerized image source by selection of specific gray levels from which the perimeter of the image is to be recorded. A third and very important level of data reduction takes place in

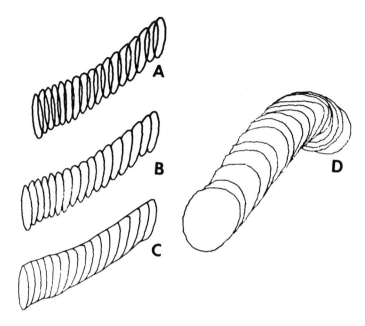

Fig. 2. Hidden-line and sideline capabilities. The examples comprise computer-aligned perimeters from the graphics display which have been obtained from the writing tablet in an interactive mode. (A) Circular profiles stacked together and rotated at about 60° on the Y axis. The overlapping ring structures produce an indecipherable image. (B) Removal of the hidden line improves the image quality and a distinct tubular structure is recognizable. By the addition of sidelining in (C), the contours are further defined. In (D), rotation of the same structure at 30° on the vertical with additional Z rotation demonstrates the structural detail which can be obtained using these software systems.

the software handling of the large number of picture points generated by the IAC. This results in a short vector display of the perimeter (Fig. 3). A further reduction of these points can be made by software through a light-pen interactive instruction (REDUCE) as shown in Fig. 3. A threshold for minimum or maximum vector length can be set in order to limit points but maintain resolution.

A second program assembles the extracted perimeters and allows for rotation of these rings (Fig. 2). Variable parameters for magnification and section separation allow a wide range of images to be reconstructed, e.g., macroscopic projection of brain surfaces or ultrastructural details of tridimensional synaptic vesicle distribution within a presynaptic terminal. Other variables such as rotation angles, object specification, and light-pen control allow considerable manipulation of the reconstruction images.

The images formed from rings are, however, not completely satisfactory

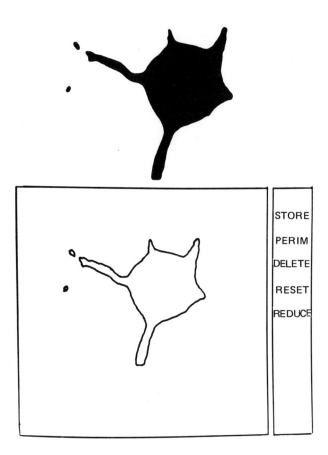

Fig. 3. *Top:* Photograph from the display of the image analysis system showing density selection which defines an optical plane of a neuronal cell body and dendrites. By changing the focus at increments, optical sectioning produces profiles throughout the dendritic tree which can be recorded for each level of the cell and processes. *Bottom:* Screen of the graphics display showing the perimeter of the optical slice which has been extracted by software from the density-selected data in the top figure. Note that even small structures are outlined. At the side of the screen are five modes which can be activated by the light pen for operator interaction with the extracted data. The PERIM instruction can be activated via light pen or via the software program to produce a perimeter trace extracting points from the selected image produced by the image analysis computer. The DELETE mode can be activated via the light pen to remove any structures which may be undesirable in the field. The REDUCE selection produces a simplification of the form by additional reduction in the points by a prescribed selection based on deviation of successive vectors.

since their overlap confuses the surface contours of the image (Fig. 2A). It is therefore necessary to process this image further to fuse the surface contours from limited data points but yet have sufficient quality to remain recognizable by the observer.

Two factors have been found to be important in producing high-quality images. First, hidden-line removal is foremost in order to unambiguously describe the contours formed by objects, especially when the rings (pages) are very close together (Figs. 2 and 4). Hidden-line removal is practical with a medium-sized laboratory computer. A simple algorithm involving a search for points where the ring will cross the pathway of an adjacent ring structure eliminates the portion which is in the back part of the field (Fig. 2). The complexity of this search increases with the complexity of the structure and the angle with which it is rotated.

Hidden-line removal is effective in most objects when the rings are sufficiently close and the viewing angle is in the range of $45°$ (Figs. 2D and 4). When looking at the rings from the side or from the end, the image is not complete. In order to overcome this problem, a second image-processing is necessary to provide a perimeter in the plane of view (sidelining) (Fig. 2C). As in the previous case, the algorithm necessary for the sidelining procedure can be developed at a relatively simple level if the image is not too complex. Otherwise, more elaborate algorithms have to be utilized in order to properly interconnect the rings at the perimeter of the object in a given perspective when multiple rings occur at the same page level (e.g., branches) or the surface is very irregular (e.g., folds).

2.2.2b. Input Methods for Branched Structures. The recording of axial coordinates of tree structures for reconstruction by a pattern of vectors is one of the most commonly utilized approaches to reconstruction of neuronal form. This method gives length and position of the processes in space as well as including information on diameter. With the input system described here, dendritic trees can be recorded by either perimeter extraction or vector-branching modes. Besides recording surface contours as described above, the perimeter extraction procedure can be used to define the axial coordinates of the dendritic trees.

2.3. Perimeter Extraction: Software Analysis of Axial Coordinates

Perimeters recorded from sectioned (optical or mechanical) tree structures are easily formed by simply stacking together the ring contours. The axis, diameter, and surface areas of tree structures can be extracted by software from these data. A number of software procedures are involved in order to define accurately the tree structures from the various processes and to identify

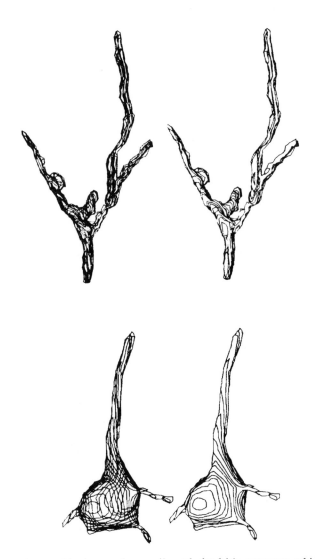

Fig. 4. Computer graphic images from cells and dendritic processes which have been recorded by the automatic perimeter extraction method. These were obtained by optical sectioning through Golgi-impregnated neurons and processes. On the left, both top and bottom, are the complete rings which form the surface contours that are rotated at approximately 45° on the Y axis. The images on the right show considerably more detail and depth as the result of hidden-line removal in the rotation program.

branching points as well as terminals. The overall advantage is that cells can be automatically recorded and analysis of the data can be tailored at the software level for the type of information about structures desired.

2.4. Interactive Vector-Branching System

The other approach to tridimensional reconstruction of tree structures consists of recording of axial coordinates for all vectors which describe the tree. Tree structures can be recorded by combined optical sectioning and page mode in the same operation. This requires that information about the points recorded be listed for each of the three coordinates. Furthermore, each point must be identified as belonging to at least one of five categories: (1) origin (usually the soma), (2) connectors (point of deflection), (3) branches, (4) terminals, and (5) interpage connectors (cut ends). Other information such as diameter, compartmentalization, and structure identification can be added.

An interactive approach is effective and has been utilized in a number of applications (Hillman *et al.*, 1974; Lindsay and Scheibel, 1974; Llinás and Hillman, 1975; Wann *et al.*, 1973). The system described here employs an interactive dual-screen input system (Fig. 1). One unit serves as the high-resolution image display and the other is the PDP-15 graphics display terminal. The image is projected via a scanner from the microscope onto the video of the IAC, while the second screen serves to specify the vectors from points indicated by the operator. A dual cursor system (Fig. 1) guided by the spark pen through a writing tablet serves to locate the appropriate points on the Quantimet image display and simultaneously record them on the graphics display. Both cursors move in unison. On the graphics screen a two-dimensional outline of the branching tree is formed by displaying the points which connect vectors to succeeding points.

The cursor on the graphics screen can also be used to localise points which have been completed by referring to the image screen. In addition, the graphics cursor is used to activate a section of the graphics screen near the base (see Fig. 6) having a specific set of instructions necessary for interactive input. Such instructions are basically labels which indicate compartments for components of the dendritic tree or axon as well as identify specific structures. In addition, other instructions include backup, shifting the field, acceptance of a dendritic tree as being complete, and completion of an entire input sequence (see Fig. 6).

In working with these systems, it has been found that high resolution in the X, Y and Z axes is essential for high-quality reconstructed images. In the Z coordinate, this is best achieved by using high magnifications and large numerical aperture lenses in order to achieve a small depth of focus. In order to quantify the Z coordinate during optical sectioning, the voltage derived from a battery through a potentiometer coupled to the fine-focus vernier is fed directly to one of the A/D converter channels. The use of an image projection system restricts the depth of field and yields precise Z coordinates to less than 0.5 μm.

The cursor system described above allows very precise specification of the X, Y coordinates via the writing tablet's spark pen (see hardware system) (Fig. 1). A matrix of as many as a million points (1000 x 1000) may be utilized on this tablet. The Quantimet, utilized in conjunction with this writing tablet and having itself 500,000 picture points, has an X, Y resolution that is less than 0.2 μm at maximum standard magnification (100 x oil).

This particular system has definite advantages over that used, for example, by Wann *et al.* (1973), where the stage is moved in order to place the structure to be recorded into register at a central marker. In our case, we find that moving the marker over the structure is much faster. A similar approach has been used by Lindsay and Scheibel (1974). In addition, the dendritic-following operation, which is executed via a large video image, is easier when the object to be followed remains stationary.

In recording the Z coordinate, the material used is the prime determinant for establishing the mode of data acquisition. If the sections are thin (i.e., less than the diameter of the processes being recorded), the thickness of the section determines the Z axis. On the other hand, if the section is thicker than the object being recorded, optical sectioning is used to determine the levels for coordinates of the process as well as the branch points which may occur within the section. Thus a combined page and optical-sectioning system is utilized.

In Golgi preparations, the processes are followed for great distances by recording the Z axis using the focal plane (optical sectioning). Additional pages are recorded by indicating cut terminals. When fluorescent dye injected cells are utilized, thinner sections are required for purely technical reasons (see Kater *et al.*, 1973). These sections are nevertheless thicker than the depth of focus of the oil immersion lens and thus contain information on branching and terminals.

In practice, the above method offers a rather straightforward way to computerize images. The program is stored on magnetic tape and can be easily loaded in a 250 K word fixed-head disk from which it can be rapidly accessed from core. A storage display is used in the setup procedure to guide the operator. Statements are indicated on the storage scope and addressed via the teletype. The format for this procedure is illustrated and described in Fig. 5.

The input procedure for recording branching neuronal processes usually begins at the soma or major part of the tree. First, four coordinate points for the limits of the soma are laid down (Fig. 6). A fifth point is used to localize the Z coordinate and is chosen by obtaining the sharpest focus. These points serve to locate the soma and indicate its size. After recording of the last point, a circle of the appropriate diameter appears on the screen and can be compared to the actual soma (Fig. 6).

```
• WHICH CHANNEL OF ADF16 IS THE POT ASSIGNED TO ? [FF]
*** TURN THE POT TO THE FIRST REFERENCE POSITION AND INPUT THE VALUE (MIC

      100 MICRON = 817

    DO YOU LIKE THIS ?  ("1" OR "0")
** I NEED ANOTHER REFERENCE POSITION

      5 MICRON = 622

    DO YOU LIKE THIS ?  ("1" OR "0")

  SCALE (100 MICRON = XXXX MILLIMETER) ?  [FF]
• INPUT THE VALUE OF THRESHOLD FOR (X,Y)  [FF]
• IS TER-COMP1 LEGAL ?  ("1" OR "0")
• WANT TO SPECIFY SOMA NOW ?  ("1" OR "0")
** INPUT FOUR POINTS (X,Y) FROM WRITING TABLET
** ADJUST THE FOCUS(Z) TO SOMA AND HIT ANY (X,Y) ON WRITING TABLET

    SOMA:   589  561  161   98

    DO YOU LIKE THIS SOMA ?  ("1" OR "0")
```

Fig. 5. Computer printout of the interactive statements for setting up the branching tree interactive-input mode. After assigning the A/D converter channel, two reference points are digitized for the Z axis and the converter output is displayed in micrometers. Then the magnification is entered in micrometers per millimeter. The threshold value for maximum length of vectors can be determined in order to limit vector length and thus improve the recording quality. In line 10, a terminal in compartment 1 can be designated as an illegal procedure. In those cases where compartment 1 processes have distal portions which are always of another type, the operator is forced to make this distinction. The remainder of statements relate to the position of the soma which appears on the screen as seen in Fig. 6.

D. E. Hillman et al.

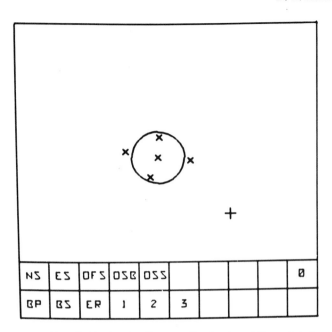

Fig. 6. PDP-15 graphics display showing the recording frame and five points for a soma. The circle represents the diameter extrapolated from the data and can be matched to the soma for size and position. These instructions are activated by using the spark-pen-guided cursor also in the circle.

In order to record dendritic tree structure, the soma or arbitrary point is visualized on the display and the initial point of origin is brought into focus by foot-pedal control to the fine-focus vernier. The spark pen on the writing tablet serves as a "joy stick" to move the cursor over the focused point of origin to be recorded and the contact switch at the spark pen is activated. This transfers the X and Y coordinates for each point into memory. The same instruction reads the Z coordinate value extrapolated from the calibration values entered at the beginning of the recording. Recorded X, Y, and Z coordinates are identified by one of five foot pedals: (1) origin, (2) connector, (3) branch, (4) terminals, and (5) interpage connectors. Following the establishment of the initial coordinates, subsequent points are recorded in a similar manner via the appropriate instruction pedal.

Connectors serve to change the direction of the vectors as the branch deviates from a straight line in any of the axes. The axis of the structure is effectively followed to each of its terminals (Fig. 7). At branching points, a cross is left on the graphic screen to guide the operator back to the unfilled branches. When a terminal is filled, the last branch recorded becomes the next point of the tree to be completed. The cross marking this branching point is intermittently

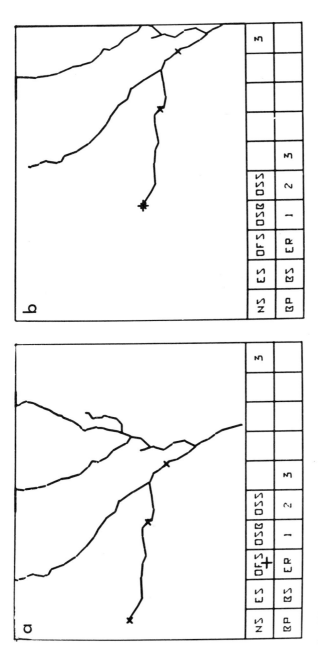

Fig. 7. Shifting of the specimen stage for objects larger than the microscopic field. Since high magnification is needed in order to obtain good resolution of the image, the stage is moved to follow branches for great distances. The offset is instructed by activating one of the three blocks OFS, OSB, or OSS. The OFS instruction is used to indicate any desired point to be shifted to any specified region of the screen. At the top, the OSB (offset branch) is activated, which displaces the graphics image so that the last-recorded branch point (leftmost cross) is shifted to the center of the screen as is shown in the lower field. At the same time, the microscope stage is automatically shifted in a similar manner to match this recording point. The OSS shifts the soma point of origin for the tree being recorded back to the center of the screen.

activated to call attention to the site (Fig. 7). If this subsequent point is actually out of the field, it is automatically returned to the center of the display by the X- and Y-axis drive motors. Those points which leave the page (section) are specified by a separate instruction (interpage connector) and thus can be used to compile the tree from component pages.

The acquisition sequence can be interrupted at any time during the recording. This allows the field to be recentered on the display as the branch is being traced (Fig. 7). By using the spark-pen-guided cursor to activate the instruction square (OFS) at the base of the graphics display (Figs. 5–7), the shift is implemented. The cursor is used to establish a reference point on the image and then the stage is shifted. The same area of the image is again recorded at its new location and the recording process is continued.

Other sequences such as centering the soma OSS or centering the current branch point OSB may also be called with a similar selection design at the base of the screen. Automatic shifting can be activated for a standard displacement in any of the four directions. A single instruction activates the stage and shifts the graphics screen. After completion of a terminal or interpage connector, the stage is automatically moved to the next branch point, or in the case where all branches are filled it is returned back to the point of origin.

Identifications of dendritic or axonic components are placed in compartments by labeling the appropriate coordinates. Before the recording procedure is initiated, one of the "storage compartments" must be activated and then subsequently changed when a different part of the tree is being followed (Fig. 7). This allows labeling of the distinctive features of neuronal trees, e.g., spiny branchlets, main parts of dendritic trees, and axons.

Since errors may be introduced, point-by-point backup has been implemented by cursor activation of the BP square (Fig. 7) at the base of the screen. This allows vectors to be removed, one at a time, with subsequent reappearance of the branch-point crosses. Rapid erasing can also be carried out by activation of the backup segment (BS) or alternatively the entire input may be erased (ER). Upon completion of a dendritic tree (i.e., when all terminals have been filled), the tree is intermittently blinked on the graphics screen to signal the end of the computing process. The completed dendritic tree is checked and then accepted by activation of the NS square (Fig. 7). Recording of other trees related to the cell is carried out following similar procedures. When all of the dendritic trees of a cell are completed, the ES instruction square is activated to signal the completion of the input.

The recorded data consist of a table of coordinates and labels specifying their type and compartment; diameter information can also be entered. The data are then placed on either paper punch tape or disk. Interpage connections in any section can be treated as terminals for the rotation program or can be used to further complete the table for the entire cell by recording subsequent pages.

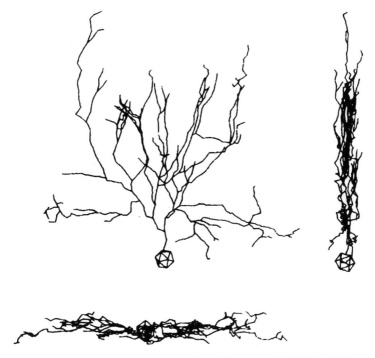

Fig. 8. Pigeon Purkinje cell by the interactive branching-tree method. The cell is rotated to show its appearance in the three Cartesian coordinate systems.

Interpage terminals are used to align the subsequent pages and join the processes.

These data may then be displayed in the image rotation mode and interacted on the graphics display as described by Llinás and Hillman (1975) (Fig. 8). When a statistically significant number of cells has been analyzed, the quantitative subroutines may be utilized to extract statistical morphological parameters, as has been done in studies by Hillman *et al.* (1974), Lindsay and Scheibel (1974), Llinás and Hillman (1975), and Wann *et al.* (1973).

3. References

Born, G., 1883, Die Plattenmodelliermethode, *Arch. Mikrosk. Anat.* **22**:584–599.

Coleman, P. D., West, M. J., and Wyss, U. R., 1973, Computer-aided quantitative neuro-anatomy, in: *Digital Computers in the Behavioral Laboratory* (B. Weiss, ed.), pp. 379–426, Appleton-Century-Crofts, New York.

Conradi, S., 1969, Observations on ultrastructure of axon hillock and initial axon segment of lumbosacral motoneurons in cat, *Acta Physiol. Scand. Suppl.* **332**: 65–84.

Garvey, C. F., Young, J. H., Jr., Coleman, P. D., and Simon, W., 1973, Automated three-dimensional dendrite tracking system, *EEG Clin. Neurophysiol.* **35**:199–204.

Glaser, E. M., and Van der Loos, H., 1965, A semi-automatic computer–microscope for the analysis of neuronal morphology, *IEEE Trans. Biomed. Eng.* **12**:22–31.

Golgi, C., 1873, Sulla struttura della sostanza grigia del cervello, *Gas. Med. Lomb.* **33**:244–246.

Hillman, D. E., Chujo, M., and Llinás, R., 1974, Quantitative computer analysis of the morphology of cerebellar neurons. I. Granule cells, *Anat. Rec.* **178**:375.

Kater, S. B., and Nicholson, C., 1973, *Intracellular Staining in Neurobiology*, Springer-Verlag, New York.

Kater, S. B., Nicholson, C., and Davis, W. J., 1973, A guide to intracellular staining techniques, in: *Intracellular Staining in Neurobiology* (S. B. Kater and C. Nicholson, eds.), pp. 307–352, Springer-Verlag, New York.

Levinthal, C., and Ware, R., 1972, Three-dimensional reconstruction from serial sections, *Nature (London)* **236**:207–210.

Levinthal, C., Macagno, E., and Tountas, C., 1974, Computer-aided reconstruction from serial sections, *Fed. Proc.* **33**:2336–2340.

Lindsay, R. D., and Scheibel, A. B., 1974, Quantitative analysis of the dendritic branching pattern of small pyramidal cells from adult rat somesthetic and visual cortex, *Exp. Neurol.* **45**:424–434.

Llinás, R., and Hillman, D. E., 1975, A multipurpose tridimensional reconstruction computer system for neuroanatomy, in: *Golgi Centennial Symposium Proceedings* (M. Santini, ed.), pp. 519–528, Raven Press, New York.

Murphey, R. K., 1973, Characterization of an insect neuron which cannot be visualized *in situ*, in: *Intracellular Staining in Neurobiology* (S. B. Kater and C. Nicholson, eds.), pp. 135–150, Springer-Verlag, New York.

Pitman, R. M., Tweedle, C. D., Cohen, M. J., 1973, The form of nerve cells: Determination by cobalt impregnation, in: *Intracellular Staining in Neurobiology* (S. B. Kater and C. Nicholson, eds.), pp. 83–97, Springer-Verlag, New York.

Reddy, D. R., Davis, W. J., Ohlander, R. B., and Bihary, D. J., 1973, Computer analysis of neuronal structure, in: *Intracellular Staining in Neurobiology* (S. B. Kater and C. Nicholson, eds.), pp. 227–253, Springer-Verlag, New York.

Selverston, A. I., 1973, The use of intracellular dye injections in the study of small neural networks, in: *Intracellular Staining in Neurobiology* (S. B. Kater and C. Nicholson, eds.), pp. 255–280, Springer-Verlag, New York.

Smith, R., Gall, C., Deadwyler, S., and Lynch, G., 1974, Dendritic transport of horseradish peroxidase *in vivo* and *in vitro*, in: *Fourth Annual Meeting of the Society for Neuroscience*, pp. 77.

Wann, D. F., Woolsey, T. A., Dierker, M. L., and Cowan, W. M., 1973, An on-line digital-computer system for the semiautomatic analysis of Golgi-impregnated neurons, *IEEE Trans. Biomed. Eng.* **20**:233–247.

Willey, T. J., Schultz, R. L., and Gott, A. H., 1973, Computer graphics in three dimensions for perspective reconstruction of brain ultrastructure, *IEEE Trans. Biomed. Eng.* **20**:288–291.

5

Semiautomatic Tracking of Neuronal Processes

*Paul D. Coleman, Catherine F. Garvey,
John H. Young, and William Simon*

1. Introduction

As the morphological sciences become more quantitative and experimental, and as more subtle phenomena are explored, the development of appropriate tools becomes important to the production of quantitative data in volume. The need for quantitative morphological data has long been recognized, and quantitative study of the nervous system was emphasized over 50 years ago by S. T. Bok, whose early work is represented in a more recent volume (Bok, 1959) and developed further by Sholl (1956) in studies of the nervous system, especially dendrites. These early efforts were, however, hampered by the lack of appropriate tools and the tedious nature of the manual data-collection procedures. As a result, many early studies dealt with relatively small numbers of measures. Some consequences of this limited data base include statistical imprecision and erroneous conclusions. As a step toward overcoming these limitations, the need for automated techniques in the morphological sciences was coupled to developing electronic technology over 20 years ago by J. Z. Young in his work with Causley on the flying-spot scanner (Causley and Young, 1955). Other early flying-spot scanners and related devices were described by Friesen (1965), Lorch (1967), Mansberg and Segarra (1962), Tolles and Mansberg (1962), Kirsch *et al.* (1957), Ledley (1964), and others. More recent dendrite measurement equipment has been described by Wann *et al.* (1973), Lindsay (1971), and Garvey *et al.* (1972, 1973).

Paul D. Coleman, Catherine F. Garvey, John H. Young, and William Simon · Department of Anatomy and Division of Biomathematics, University of Rochester Medical Center, Rochester, New York 14642.

The more recent coupling of the general-purpose digital computer to image-input devices has, however, produced great advances in automated and semiautomated collection of quantitative morphological data. In general, these techniques deal with images in which the desired objects are easily detected on the basis of optical density: e.g., grains in autoradiography (Wann *et al.*, 1974), E-PTA-stained synapses in electron microscopy (West *et al.*, 1972), dendrites in Golgi-stained material (Garvey *et al.*, 1973), opaque capillaries in microfil-injected material (Weindl and Joynt, 1971), etc. Once detected, these structures may be counted and/or measured in a variety of ways.

As more sophisticated pattern-recognition techniques are applied to analysis of morphological material, it can be anticipated that the range of structures that can be studied will be broadened to include those that can be defined in terms related to shape and gray level in relatively complex ways. Such a more sophisticated pattern-recognition approach is currently being applied in our laboratory in conjunction with the Departments of Computer Science and Neurology in the recognition, typing, counting, and measuring of muscle fiber types.

Our desire to make a dendrite-tracking system that was relatively highly automated led to the requirement that data points collected through the microscope by the system be closely spaced in X, Y and Z (depth or focus level). The smaller the steps the system takes in following a dendrite, the narrower the limits of the search area for the next point, and consequently the less the probability of erroneous tracking (with certain assumptions regarding the extrapolation algorithm). The distance between successive data points is 0.8 μm in X and Y, and 0.5 μm in Z. Each point is characterized as either (1) start of a primary dendrite, (2) branch point, (3) end point passing out of plane of section (cut end), (4) end point within the plane of the section, or (5) continuation of the segment being tracked.

2. Hardware

A block diagram of the major aspects of the hardware of the system is shown in Fig. 1. The major items of equipment are a Data General 1220 computer system, a Leitz Orthoplan microscope, and an ITT Vidissector (image dissector).

The Vidissector is the device which converts the optical density information of the microscope into analog electrical signals suitable for input to the analog-to-digital (A/D) converter of the computer. When desired, the microscope may be bypassed and the Vidissector can look at larger images directly through standard lenses. Figure 2 shows a diagram of the tube which is the heart of the

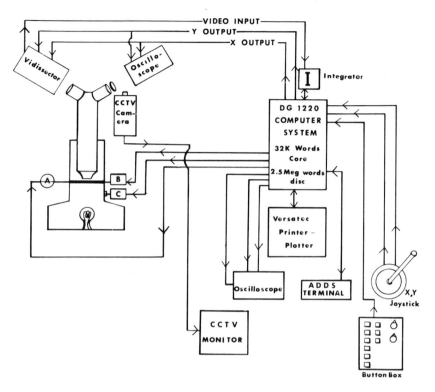

Fig. 1. Block diagram of the apparatus. The two optical paths from the two eyepieces of the microscope go to the Vidissector from one eyepiece and to the projection oscilloscope (via a lens and mirrors) from the other eyepiece. A, B, and C represent stepping motors driven by the computer which move the microscope stage in X, Y, and Z. The operator control area is located in the lower right-hand portion of the figure adjacent to the joy stick, button box, ADDS alphanumeric video terminal, and closed-circuit television monitor. I represents the integrator.

Vidissector. Light energy falling on the photo sensitive surface of the tube causes the emission of electrons which are focused and accelerated toward the anode. The passage of most of these electrons to the anode is blocked by a metal plate with a small aperture (1 mil diameter in the tube in our system) which allows the electrons from only a small region of the 1-inch-diameter photosensitive surface to pass to the anode. The electrons may be deflected by voltages applied to the horizontal and vertical deflection plates of the Vidissector. Thus the deflection plates control which spatial subsample of the electrons pass through the 1-mil aperture to the anode and consequently which portion of the scene falling on the face of the Vidissector determines the output of the Vidissector. The Vidissector may be considered a spatially selective PMT (photomultiplier tube)

Photo-sensitive
Surface   Diaphragm

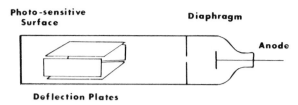

Anode

Deflection Plates

Fig. 2. Drawing illustrating the principle of operation of an image dissector tube as described in the text. The focus coil and electron multiplier elements have been omitted for the sake of clarity. (A more detailed description, as well as performance characteristics, may be found in Technical Note 112 from the Electron Tube Division, Tube and Sensor Laboratories, ITT, 3700 East Pontiac St., Ft. Wayne, Indiana 46803.)

with random access to any X, Y location within the total field covered by the Vidissector. The computer determines (through two D/A converters) the voltages applied to the deflection plates and consequently which portion of the image falling on the face of the Vidissector is having its optical density sampled by the system.

The output of the Vidissector is relayed to the computer through an integrator, multiplexer, and an A/D converter. The computer may therefore make decisions under program control about which location to examine next, based on what has been found at locations previously examined.

Since the photosensitive surface of the Vidissector is a non-integrating surface, its output must be integrated in a subsequent stage to obtain an adequate signal/noise ratio. The duration of the integration period is under program control. The integration period is a function of the signal/noise ratio desired, which is in turn related to the resolution required of the system. Thick dendrites give a very adequate signal/noise ratio with little or no integration of the Vidissector output (see Fig. 5). Thin dendrites would, with the same integration period, yield a density plot (see Fig. 7 for some examples) with a much poorer signal/noise ratio. They therefore require longer integration periods. In practice, with our Golgi–Cox material, we have found an integration period of 50 μsec to be adequate for the detection of the smallest dendrite or axonal branches. We use this as a fixed integration period at every point. It would be possible to write a subroutine that would integrate until a predetermined signal/noise ratio had been reached. This is being done at Washington University, St. Louis (Professor D. Wann, personal communication).

There do exist devices other than the ITT Vidissector which can randomly access picture points and read optical density at the point accessed. These alternate devices each have their own advantages and disadvantages. Technology of these devices is changing rapidly, so a comparison of specific devices does not seem warranted here. However, properties that might well be compared include storage vs. nonstorage surfaces, resolution, nondestructive readout, access time, and random vs. nonrandom access to picture points.

When a dendrite being tracked passes out of the microscope field, the X, Y stage-stepping motors move the stage, under computer control, so that the dendrite being tracked is brought back into the field. X, Y coordinates being explored by the Vidissector are displaced by an amount equal to the stage displacement so that tracking resumes at the proper place.

As tracking progresses, the dendrite is automatically kept in focus by computer control of a stepping motor attached to the fine-focus control of the microscope. Steps of this motor provide the Z coordinate aspect of the X, Y, Z coordinate record of the dendrite.

During tracking, a degree of operator interaction with the system may take place through (1) the joy stick, which is used to provide operator input of X, Y information, and (2) the "button box," which is used to answer queries issued by the computer, provides for operator intervention in case of error, allows operator input of Z information and direction information at certain intervention points, etc. The functions of the "button box" are shown in Fig. 3.

Since the tracking algorithm requires some degree of operator interaction with the system, it is essential that the operator know at all times what local regions the system is exploring and what decisions the system is making about these local regions. This is made possible in large part by the "projection" oscilloscope indicated in Fig. 1.

The light path through one eyepiece of the microscope (i.e., light source—substage condenser-slide—objective—right eyepiece) is directed by a set of lenses and mirrors onto the face of the projection oscilloscope so that the microscope field is imaged on the face of the projection oscilloscope. (Note that the image formed by the left eyepiece falls on the Vidissector.) This optical path is arranged to correspond to the optical path from the microscope to the Vidissector in such a way that the image falling on the projection oscilloscope corresponds point to point with the image falling on the Vidissector face. In other words, the image falling on the 5-inch CRT of the projection oscilloscope is an enlarged version of the image falling on the 1-inch Vidissector face, and the focus is equivalent in both images.

In addition, the horizontal and vertical deflection plates of the projection oscilloscope are in parallel with the horizontal and vertical deflection plates of the Vidissector. The horizontal and vertical gain and position controls of the projection oscilloscope are adjusted so that the X, Y position of the beam of the oscilloscope is an exactly scaled (in proportion to the ratio of image sizes falling on the Vidissector and projection oscilloscope) replica of X, Y coordinates being sent to the Vidissector by the computer for sampling of optical density. Thus, by looking at the position of the oscilloscope beam with respect to the optical image projected onto the face of the projection oscilloscope, the operator knows exactly what X, Y (and Z) location of the microscope field is currently being examined by the computer.

This knowledge enables the operator to monitor the accuracy of the

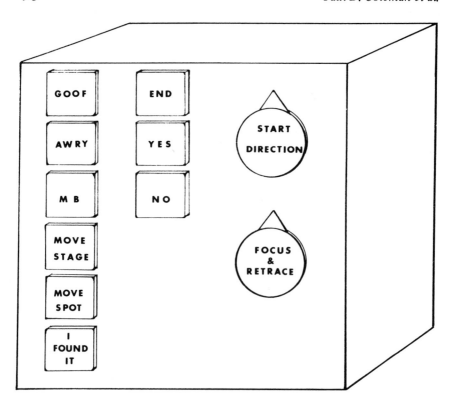

Fig. 3. "Button box" controls. If an inappropriate button is pushed by accident, the GOOF button will return the program to where it was just before the inappropriate button was pushed. The operation of the MB (MISSED BRANCH) and AWRY buttons is described in the text. The MOVE STAGE and MOVE SPOT buttons determine whether the joy stick moves the microscope stage in X and Y (by means of the stepping motors) or whether it moves the beam of the projection oscilloscope, thereby telling the Vidissector where to "look" within the microscope field. The I FOUND IT button signifies to the computer that the operator has found a cell body, or dendrite beginning, or starting direction or branch point (operator defined). The END button signifies that all dendrites of a cell have been identified, all cells for the current batch have been found, operator intervention has ended, or the operator has declared a dendrite ending. The upper right potentiometer is used to signify starting directions and the lower right potentiometer is used for operator focus and operator control of retrace after MISSED BRANCH or TRACKING AWRY have been pushed.

tracking by the system, to interrupt and correct when tracking becomes inaccurate, and to respond to queries from the system such as those requesting confirmation of branch points, endings, etc. (described in more detail below).

Once the dendritic tree of a single cell has been completely tracked, the tree is displayed on the oscilloscope and/or a Versatec printer-plotter. Numerical information about the tree is also printed out on the Versatec or a Teletype, as described below.

3. Software

To use the system to track dendrites, the operator, viewing the back-projected image of the microscope field on the projection oscilloscope, selects a cell whose dendrites are to be measured. This is done by moving the microscope stage by means of the joystick—computer—stage-stepping motors hardware subsystem. At the same time, he operator can alter focus (in 0.5-μm steps) by means of the (button box) potentiometer—computer—fine-focus stepping motor subsystem. Once a cell to be measured has been identified, the operator focuses it sharply and positions the projection oscilloscope beam in the center of the cell using the joy stick. The operator then pushes the button I FOUND IT thereby informing the computer of the X, Y, and Z coordinates to be taken as the cell center. The computer asks for cell identification information (see Table I), after which the operator is free to identify additional cells if desired.

Once a sequence of cells has been identified, the computer returns the stage to the first cell identified and asks the operator to identify primary dendrites (by means of the joy stick and focusing potentiometer) and the direction of initial travel of the first dendrite. The operator provides this last information using the direction potentiometer mounted in the button box. This potentiometer swings the beam of the projection oscilloscope around clock positions. When a dendrite's initial direction has been found, the operator presses the I FOUND IT button. Once all dendrites of a cell have been identified, the operator indicates this to the computer by pushing the button END.

The computer will then track the first-identified dendrite of the first cell and move automatically to the next-identified dendrite. Once the dendrites of one cell have been tracked, the computer moves to the next cell, tracking the dendrites of each cell until all previously selected cells have been tracked.

3.1. Tracking

The initial event in computer tracking, once operator initialization has been completed, is the sampling of light intensities (densities) on a semicircle which has as its center the starting point of a dendrite (indicated by the operator), with the midpoint on the circumference determined by the angular position indicated by the operator as the initial direction of tracking. The darkest and lightest light levels seen by the Vidissector on this semicircle are determined and a "threshold" level is defined as the average of these two levels. Any light level (density) darker than threshold is considered to represent a stained element; any density lighter than threshold is considered to be noise, except at branch regions. In order to compensate for local variations in density of illumination or background staining, "threshold" is adjusted after each 10 μm of tracking using essentially this same procedure.

The dendrite-tracking algorithm is based on examination of the density plot formed as the Vidissector examines a series of points that lie on an arc across a dendrite. Figure 4 shows a portion of a dendrite with a sequence of points whose optical density is examined. A plot of optical density (i.e., Vidissector output) as a function of position on the scanning arc is shown in Fig. 5. The arc position(s) showing the greatest optical density is, of course, an indication of the angular position of the dendrite in a polar coordinate system, and forms the basis for the decision as to where to start the next search arc. Note the sequence in which points on the search arc are explored as shown in Fig. 4. The first search point is at the X, Y coordinate predicted to be the center of the dendrite based on the last known position of the dendrite, assuming that the dendrite will continue in a line that will deviate no more than one point from a straight line. Points are searched in the sequence shown until a set of points satisfying threshold is found (additionally, a fixed number of points beyond threshold at each side of the arc are examined in order to search for possible branchings) or until a limit in number of points to be searched has been reached without finding any points satisfying the threshold criterion. In this latter case, and end is assumed and procedures follow which are described below in more detail.

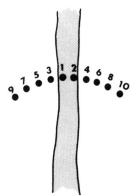

Fig. 4. Diagram illustrating the sampling sequence along an arc across a dendrite. The numbers indicate the sequence in which points are sampled.

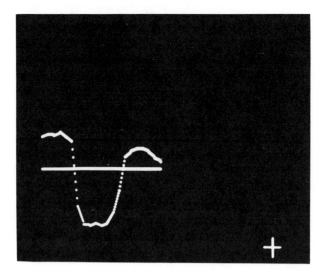

Fig. 5. Density plot (i.e., sampling of Vidissector output) obtained from examination of a series of points across a thick dendrite. The straight line is a representation of the computer-determined threshold. A "+" or "−" in the lower right indicates the direction of movement (up or down) last taken by the focus-stepping motor.

3.2. Branch Detection

If a double dip is found in the density plot of one search arc, the computer infers the class of structures illustrated in Fig. 6 and queries the operator BRANCH? A sampling of density plots which were considered to represent branch regions is shown in Fig. 7. It can be seen that a variety of forms of density plots may be considered to represent branch regions.

The computer classifies a density plot as representing a possible branch pattern if, in addition to the single dip of an unbranched dendrite, two conditions are satisfied: (1) the slope of the density plot has changed sign and this new slope sign has been maintained for more than two consecutive points on the density plot, and (2) the amplitude of this changed slope exceeds an arbitrarily defined magnitude. This arbitrarily defined magnitude was defined on the basis of empirical trials.

If branch regions were always limited to the X, Y plane, with both branches emerging along the same focus level, detection of branchings would be a relatively simple problem. However, immediately after a branch point one branch may go in one Z direction, the other branch in the opposite Z direction. Thus it is necessary to examine density plots for branch activity (as shown in Fig. 7) as a function of focus level.

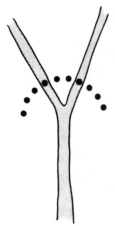

Fig. 6. Diagram illustrating the sampling of points at a branch region.

Once a branch pattern has been found in the density plot at any focus level at a particular arc position, eight focus levels around that level are explored. If a branch pattern is found at N of these eight focus levels, then a branch point is considered to have been defined. Empirical trials have shown $N = 5$ to be optimal. This criterion tends to err in the direction of giving more false positives (perhaps due to dendritic spines) than false negatives. We adopted this strategy because it is relatively less time consuming for the operator to deal with a false positive (by pushing the NO button in response to a BRANCH? query) than it is to deal with a missed branch (discussed in Section 3.5).

Once a branching has been determined, the computer arbitrarily follows one of the branches. The branch followed is usually the one giving the larger light—dark difference at the focus level at which the branch decision was reached. As the tracking progresses, successive branch points are identified and their locations are stored in a stack, or list, of branch-point coordinates.

Once the end of a dendrite has been detected, as described below, the computer automatically returns to the most recent unfilled branch region (the most recently defined branch point). A row of dots is displayed along the branch that was tracked and the operator is asked to indicate the starting direction of the untracked branch. This is done in the same way that starting direction of the primary dendrite is indicated. Tracking will then proceed as before until the end of another dendrite is detected. The computer works its way in this manner through the stack (or list) of branch regions until the most proximal (to the cell body) branch has been filled. The computer then proceeds automatically to the next-identified primary dendrite and requests information about starting direction as previously described.

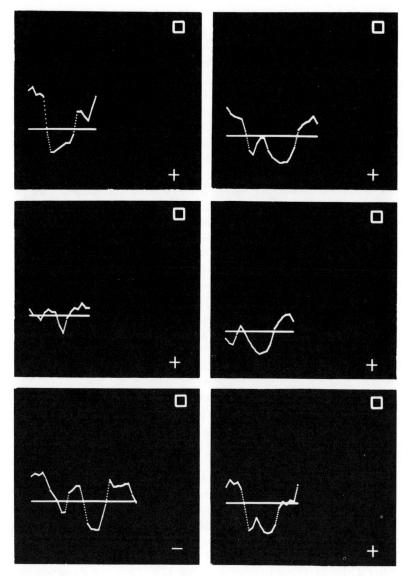

Fig. 7. Examples of density plots obtained at branch regions. All density plots are at the same horizontal and vertical gain. Same conventions as in Fig. 5. In addition, the square in the upper right indicates that the computer has decided that the density plot shown is representative of a branch region. In each density plot, amplitude differences between the dips representing the two branches are a reflection of differences in focal plane or width of the branches. The various density plots represent regions in which dendrite thicknesses are both thick and thin. Note that in regions of thick dendrites (broader, deeper dips) the density plots extend over more points (greater horizontal extent) as a consequence of this greater thickness.

3.3. Automatic Focusing

As a dendrite meanders through X and Y within the thick (200 μm) sections cut for study of Golgi–Cox stained material, its variations in the Z dimension (focus level) are considerable. For automated tracking to be possible, as well as to collect three-dimensional information, the dendrite being tracked must be kept in extremely precise focus. This is accomplished by repeated search arcs over the same set of X, Y coordinates as the computer varies the microscope fine focus by means of the computer-controlled stepping motor attached to the microscope fine-focus control. Thus an arc is probed at one focus level, the focus level is changed (by 0.5 μm), and the same X, Y coordinates are probed at the new focus level. These data are analyzed in two ways: (1) light and dark peaks are analyzed to detect branch points, and (2) three points on either side of the darkest point of the original arc are investigated. If the density at any of these three points gets darker than the initial darkest point, a new ("better") focus is considered found.

Two focusing steps, in each direction, up and down, are made. If a better focus (i.e., greater density) is found in either direction, more focusing steps in that direction are tried. Otherwise, the original focus position is restored. A set of density plots illustrating a focus search is shown in Fig. 8.

3.4. End Detection

At the end of a dendrite, no points exceeding threshold are found within the limits of the search region, and the computer queries END? At this time, the operator can search through focus levels by means of the focus potentiometer. The operator has the additional option of forcing a change in the direction of tracking by means of the direction potentiometer. The operator may respond to the END? query by pushing the NO button, changing focus and forcing a new tracking direction. Alternatively, if an end has indeed been found, the operator will push the YES button. The computer will then respond with the query CUT END? (i.e., "Did the dendrite pass out of the plane of section."), to which the operator responds by pushing the YES or NO button.

After the end of the last unfilled branch of a cell has been reached, the computer writes on a disk a record of all the X, Y, Z points tracked, along with the experiment and cell identification information illustrated in Tables I and II. If more than one cell has been identified for tracking, the computer automatically moves the stage in X, Y, and Z to the first dendrite to be tracked of the next cell selected and requests a starting direction.

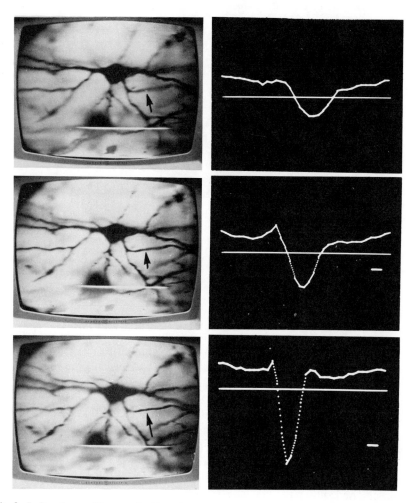

Fig. 8. Left column: Picture of video display of microscope field. Arrows indicate region being focused. The scanning arc does not appear because it was too brief to be captured on film. Right column: Density plots as a function of focus adjustments. Top picture: initially poor focus in region under consideration. Middle picture: Computer has moved the focus-stepping motor five steps down and found the dip in the density plot to become greater. Video display shows improved focus at arrow. Bottom picture: Computer has moved focus-stepping motor nine steps down and determined that additional steps do not increase the dip in the density plot. Focus is optimal.

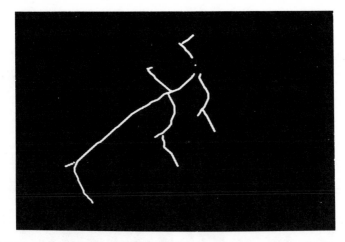

Fig. 9. Oscilloscope display of X and Y coordinates of a stellate cell. A cell with a relatively simple dendritic tree was chosen for ease of comparison with the quantitative data in Tables I, II, and III. There are three primary dendrites arising from the cell body. The dot near the origin of the primary dendrites represents the center of the cell body as determined by the operator.

3.5. Error Correction

If the computer tracking strays away from the dendrite being tracked, the operator pushes the button (tracking) AWRY. Computer tracking then halts and the operator can initiate and control a retrace (by means of the focus-retrace potentiometer on the button box) through the list of X, Y, Z coordinates stored since the last branch point. This retrace is also displayed on the projection oscilloscope. When the point is reached at which tracking first went awry, the operator pushes the button END. The coordinates that have been retraced are then deleted from the records. The operator may then manually track over the problem region using the joy stick and focus knob. Once the problem region has been traversed, the operator pushes END again, the computer asks for a starting direction, and automatic tracking is resumed. In practice, this procedure is necessary about once or twice for the average cell in cerebral cortex.

If a branch point is passed without being identified, the operator pushes the button MB (MISSED BRANCH). Tracking halts, and retrace is controlled by the operator with the focus-retrace potentiometer. When the missed branch point is reached, the operator pushes the button I FOUND IT. The system then resumes tracking at the place at which the operator pushed the MISSED BRANCH button. The operator-identified branch point is added to the list of unfilled branch regions as though it had been a computer-identified branch point. In practice, this operation is required about three or four times for the average cell in cerebral cortex.

Table I. Orders and Lengths of Dendrite Segments for the Cell Shown in Fig. 9[a]

SLIDE IDENTIFICATION:
   TODAY'S DATE = 3/14/76
   OPERATOR = PDC
   STUDY = DEM
   EXPERIMENTAL GROUP = CNTRL
   ANIMAL NUMBER = 17
   SLIDE NUMBER = 8
CELL IDENTIFICATION:
   BRAIN REGION = VI
   LAYER = 4
   CELL TYPE = STEL
   CELL NUMBER = 53

DENDRITE #1

POSITION	SEGMENT LENGTH	DISTANCE FROM CENTER	
0	+.1591497E+02	+.2191680E+02	
01	+.1003726E+02	+.3116176E+02	
00	+.2401778E+02	+.3710234E+02	

DENDRITE #2

POSITION	SEGMENT LENGTH	DISTANCE FROM CENTER	
0	+.4020108E+02	+.4469203E+02	
01	+.1589092E+02	+.5690627E+02	
00	+.2523822E+02	+.7478798E+02	

DENDRITE #3

POSITION	SEGMENT LENGTH	DISTANCE FROM CENTER	
0	+.3005125E+02	+.3208250E+02	
00	+.4234185E+01	+.3551387E+02	
001	+.1464493E+03	+.1540201E+03	
0010	+.5381937E+02	+.1796916E+03	
0011	+.1003246E+02	+.1696339E+03	
000	+.5104283E+02	+.7402213E+02	
0001	+.2197744E+02	+.8751623E+02	
0000	+.3834222E+02	+.1092398E+03	
01	+.2940798E+02	+.4272128E+02	
011	+.7160456E+01	+.4610066E+02	CUT END
010	+.1044754E+02	+.4107580E+02	

[a]Identification information is part of the record that is maintained for each cell throughout processing. Dendrite 1 is the first dendrite identified on that cell by the operator. Dendrites 2 and 3 are clockwise around the cell body. Under the POSITION column, segments with one digit represent primary (first-order) dendrites. Segments with two digits represent daughter segments (i.e., second-order dendrites), etc. The numbering of daughter segments always indicates which branch was the parent and whether the daughter segment was the right or left segment. For example, segment 001 originated from segment 00 and was the left daughter segment. The column labeled SEGMENT LENGTH indicates the distance from the start to the end (whether by branching or ending) of the segment specified. Length is in micrometers and includes all meanderings of the dendrite, rather than being the straight line from the start of the segment to its end. The column labeled DISTANCE FROM CENTER indicates the straight-line distance (in three dimensions) from the center of the cell body to the end of the segment. All segments which have been cut in the sectioning process are indicated by CUT END. Segments without this comment have ended within the section.

Paul D. Coleman et al.

Table II. Three-Dimensional Branching Angles of Dendrites for the Cell Shown in Fig. 9[a]

SLIDE IDENTIFICATION:
   TODAY'S DATE = 3/14/76
   OPERATOR = PDC
   STUDY = DEM
   EXPERIMENTAL GROUP = CNTRL
   ANIMAL NUMBER = 17
   SLIDE NUMBER = 8
CELL IDENTIFICATION:
   BRAIN REGION = VI
   LAYER = 4
   CELL TYPE = STEL
   CELL NUMBER = 53

DENDRITE #1

ORDER	NEAR ANGLE	FARANGLE (COS#)	CAT
1	+.5400887e+00	+.3529317E+00	3
	SIDE ANGLES	−.9894042E+00	
		−.4665911E+00	

DENDRITE #2

ORDER	NEAR ANGLE	FAR ANGLE (COS#)	CAT
1	+.8004016E+00	+.9639621E+00	3
	SIDE ANGLES	−.9670889E+00	
		−.9996810E+00	

DENDRITE #3

ORDER	NEAR ANGLE	FAR ANGLE (COS#)	CAT
1	+.8572564E+00	+.5177629E+00	1
	SIDE ANGLES	−.9225699E+00	
		−.1516204E+00	
2	+.5817549E+00	+.7371101E+00	1
	SIDE ANGLES	−.9355770E+00	
		−.4839602E+00	
3	+.9164054E+00	+.2898926E+00	3
	SIDE ANGLES	−.4914248E+00	
		−.9649224E+00	
3	+.7917836E+00	+.3455325E+00	3
	SIDE ANGLES	−.9397404E+00	
		+.3681108E−01	
2	+.6610024E+00	+.6095558E+00	4
	SIDE ANGLES	−.8355220E+00	
		−.8677272E+00	

---

[a]In the column ORDER, 1 indicates the angle formed by the two daughter branches of a first-order dendrite, etc. NEAR ANGLE is the angle formed by the branches when the angle is taken from the branch point to a position 2 μm out each branch. FAR ANGLE is taken from the branch point to a position 10 μm (or the closest distance to 10 μm in the case of short segments) out each branch. The SIDE ANGLES are the angles formed between each of the daughter branches and the parent branch. The CAT column categorizes the angles as follows: 1, intermediate branches; 2 terminal branches, both cut: 3 terminal branches, neither cut; 4, terminal branches, one cut. Note: all angles are solid angles.

Table III. Computer Output from Dendrite Orientation Program for Cell Shown in Fig. 9[a]

USING SOMA CENTER AS ORIGIN					
IN 3 DIMENSIONS...					
AXIS 1 MAGNITUDE = 0.180E	7,	RELATIVE MAGNITUDE = 0.600E			2
ORIENTATION = 0.637E	0	0.706E	0	0.307E	0
AXIS 2 MAGNITUDE = 0.148E	6,	RELATIVE MAGNITUDE = 0.492E			1
ORIENTATION = 0.459	0	−0.668E	0	0.584E	0
AXIS 3 MAGNITUDE = 0.301E	5,	RELATIVE MAGNITUDE = 0.100E			1
ORIENTATION = −0.618E	0	0.230E	0	0.750E	0
USING CENTER OF MASS AS ORIGIN					
IN 3 DIMENSIONS...					
AXIS 1 MAGNITUDE = 0.737E	6,	RELATIVE MAGNITUDE = 0.310E			2
ORIENTATION = 0.668E	0	0.590E	0	0.452E	0
AXIS 2 MAGNITUDE = 0.119E	6,	RELATIVE MAGNITUDE = 0.504E			1
ORIENTATION = 0.424E	0	−0.801E	0	0.420E	0
AXIS 3 MAGNITUDE = 0.237E	5,	RELATIVE MAGNITUDE = 0.999E			0
ORIENTATION = −0.611E	0	0.894E	−1	0.786E	0

[a]Principal directions of dispersion are shown for soma-centered and center-or-mass-centered coordinates. Axis magnitudes indicate amount of dispersion in orthogonal axis directions (see Brown, Chapter 10). Relative magnitudes are scaled so that the smallest dispersion is unity. Axis orientations are given by three direction cosines for each axis. Axis 1, the axis of largest magnitude, is in the direction of maximum dispersion. From its direction cosines, it is seen that the cell is most elongated in the 2 o'clock−8 o'clock direction. The other two axes show the next-smallest elongation in the orthogonal 11 o'clock−4 o'clock direction and little elongation in the Z direction. The coordinate system which is initially referred to the X, Y, and Z axes of the microscope stage may be rotated by this orientation program so that the X, Y, and Z axes are derived from brain landmarks on the slide. The orientation information then refers to known orientations within the brain.

3.6. Data Output

At the completion of tracking, a program may be called which displays the dendritic tree on an oscilloscope, where it may be manipulated and photographed. Alternatively, the tree may be drawn on a Versatec printer-plotter. Quantitative information about the dendritic tree is also printed out on the Versatec or on a Teletype. Programs currently exist to determine length and order of each dendritic branch, distance of end of segment (either by branching or ending) from the center of the cell body, three-dimensionally computed angles (both external and internal) between branches, and an analysis of elongation and orientation of the dendritic tree. This last analysis determines the best-fit set of planes to the swarm of X, Y, and Z coordinates representing the dendritic tree. This algorithm is based on earlier work of Pearson (1901) (see

Chapter 10 for a more complete exposition of this algorithm). A set of examples of the data printout from a single cell is shown in Fig. 9 and Tables I, II, and III.

These data are then typed (soon to be sent via modem) into an IBM 360/65, using APL, for more complex analyses involving large data matrices from many cells (e.g., principal component analyses).

4. Conclusions

We have constructed and programmed a system that will track cell processes of single neurons in Golgi-stained material and derive quantitative information from the tracking record. Operator participation in the tracking process is still required in the form of operator responses to simple queries from the computer, and operator intervention in the event of an incorrect move in tracking. Although operator intervention is still present, the degree of control the operator has over tracking is considerably reduced from hand tracing. As a consequence of the relatively high degree of automation, reliability is increased and the possibility of bias, although still present, is considerably reduced. We wish to emphasize here that *any* degree of operator participation in the collection of data leads to the possibility of bias in the results. It is still necessary that the data be collected blind, and, in addition, that slides from various anaimals, regions, etc., be randomly intermixed.

It currently requires on the order of 15 min (depending on the complexity of the tree) to track the processes of a single cell. The rate-limiting step in the speed of the tracking process is the human operator, for the tracking process itself—uninterrupted by any halt for operator decisions—is capable of moving at a rate of about 20 μm/sec. This rate could be increased significantly, particularly, we believe, by a more efficient focusing algorithm. However, the tracking rate would then be too fast for easy, reliable operator monitoring. The programming effort required to significantly reduce the necessity for operator monitoring and intervention appears to be extremely extensive and the resulting algorithms well might reduce tracking speed by an order of magnitude or more. We doubt that it will be feasible to completely eliminate operator monitoring, although such statements sometimes have a way of quickly being demonstrated to be incorrect.

With no program modification, but merely trivial changes in the way the operator uses the program, the system can provide the same variety of information for other structures such as axons or blood vessels, and also be used in such a way as to differentiate among portions of the dendritic tree of various cell types.

Although the tracking system described here is relatively highly automated, its major contribution to quantitative studies of neuronal processes is one that is shared with other computerized tracking systems: it gets X, Y, and Z data describing dendritic trees into a computer at a relatively rapid rate, so that these data are then easily available for quantitative analysis. Because of the decreased reliance on the operator, reliability is increased, however.

5. References

Bok, S. T., 1959, *Histonomy of the Cerebral Cortex*, Elsevier, New York.

Causley, D., and Young, J. Z., 1955, Counting and sizing of particles with the flying-spot microscope, *Nature (London)* **176**:453.

Friesen, D., 1965, A Description of the PEPR system, *DECUS Proc.,* Spring.

Garvey, C. F., Young, J., Simon, W., and Coleman, P. D., 1972, Semi-automatic dendrite tracking and focusing by computer, *Anat. Rec.* **172**:314.

Garvey, C. F., Young, J. H., Coleman, P. D., and Simon, W., 1973, Automated three-dimensional dendrite tracking system, *Electroencephalogr. Clin. Neurophysiol.* **35**:199.

Kirsch, R. A., Cahn, L., Ray, L. C., and Urban, G. H., 1957, Experiments in processing pictorial information with a digital computer, *Proc. Eastern Joint Computer Conf.* (Washington, D.C.). p. 221.

Ledley, R. S., 1964, High speed automatic analysis of biomedical pictures, *Science* **146**:216.

Lindsay, R. D., 1971, Connectivity of the cerebral cortex, doctoral dissertation, Syracuse University.

Lorch, S., 1967, Computer image processing of biological specimens, *DECUS Proc.,* Spring.

Mansberg, H. P., and Segarra, J. M., 1962, Counting of neurons by flying spot microscope, *Ann. N. Y. Acad. Sci.* **99**:309.

Pearson, K., 1901, On lines and planes of closest fit to systems of points in space, *Philosophical Magazine*, 6th ser., No. 2, July–December, p. 559.

Sholl, D. A., 1956, *The Organization of the Cerebral Cortex*, Wiley, New York.

Tolles, W. W., and Mansberg, H. P., 1962, Size and shape determination in scanning microscopy, *Ann. N. Y. Acad. Sci.* **97**:516.

Wann, D. F., Woolsey, T., Dierker, M. L., and Cowan, W. M., 1973, An on-line computer system for the semi-automatic analysis of Golgi impregnated neurons, *IEEE Trans. Biomed. Eng.* **20(4)**:233.

Wann, D. F., Price, J. L., Cowan, W. M., and Agulnek, M. A., 1974, An automated system for counting silver grains in autoradiographs, *Brain Res.* **81**:31.

Weindel, A., and Joynt, R. J. 1971, The median eminence as a circumventricular organ, in: K. M. Knigge, D. E. Scott, and A. Weindl (eds.), *Brain–Endocrine Interaction: Median Eminence: Structure and Function* (Int. Symp., Munich, 1971), pp. 280–297, Karger, Basel.

West, M. J., Coleman, P. D., and Wyss, U. R. 1972, A computerized method of determining the number of synaptic contacts in a volume of cerebral cortex, *J. Microsc.* **95**:277.

6

Online Computerized Analysis of Peripheral Nerves

R. F. Dunn, D. P. O'Leary, and W. E. Kumley

1. Introduction

The analysis of anatomical structure has been greatly aided by the increased availability of computers in the laboratory. Three-dimensional information from Golgi-impregnated neurons and their processes is particularly suited to computer-aided analysis. Another subject of interest involves the quantitative study of perimeters which characterize individual fibers comprising a nerve bundle. This includes dimensional information about axons and their myelin sheaths and statistical considerations of their numbers and size ranges, as well as their spatial distribution within the bundle. While various methods have previously been used for deriving axon diameters, the direct method of measuring diameters manually is often limited by time considerations. That is, the amount of sampling which can be completed within a reasonable time period may not be adequate as a statistically significant representation of the total nerve fiber population.

Certainly many methods exist by which quantitative information can be obtained from micrographs. One method is to draw the entire perimeter, which, while it may achieve maximum accuracy and be required of highly irregular shapes, remains time consuming. In contrast, digitization of a small number of points around the perimeter can provide sufficient resolution for measuring circular, or nearly circular, cross-sections, and speeds the rate of data entry. The

R. F. Dunn and D. P. O'Leary • Department of Surgery, UCLA School of Medicine, Los Angeles, California 90024; and Department of Otolaryngology, University of Pittsburgh School of Medicine, Pittsburgh, Pennsylvania 15213. _W. E. Kumley_ • Department of Surgery, UCLA School of Medicine, Los Angeles, California 90024.

use of particle size analyzers will certainly speed the input process, but spatial information would be difficult to obtain. Similarly, the "circle of best fit" methods (Fernand and Young, 1951; Donovan, 1967; Matthews, 1968; Matthews and Duncan, 1971; Williams and Wendell-Smith, 1960) are fairly fast, but spatial information is lost as is all possibility of changing the grouping dimensions. Stereological methods are available to estimate mean diameters (Weibel, 1973); however, these often require careful experimental design and computer-assisted analysis (e.g., see Weibel, 1973; Eisenberg *et al.*, 1974), and for these reasons might not be attractive for all applications. Another important consideration to the system detailed here is that the system functions within terms familiar to the anatomist, thereby allowing maximum operator–computer interaction with a minimum of familiarization.

The online computer-analysis system described here has been developed in response to these problems. The system is based on the use of an eight-point input algorithm for the digital storage of nerve fiber perimeters. This significantly increases the rapidity of measurements and permits computation of several numerical and statistical values in addition to information concerning the relative spatial relationships of fibers within the bundle.

2. Histological and Photographic Preparation

Specimen preparation is an important step in the analysis scheme since it forms the basis for accuracy of the input information. The necessary tissue requirements include optimum tissue preservation, proper orientation during sectioning, use of thin sections to optimize optical resolution, rigorous calibration of microscope magnification, and careful control during the photographic preparation of the final prints.

The requirements of fixation are tissue dependent in the sense that the fixative should be designed to match the osmolarity of the specific tissue under investigation (Bohman, 1974; Karlsson and Schultz, 1965; Sjöstrand, 1967), and it should be delivered with a minimum lapse of postmortem time. The fixation of elasmobranch tissue is further complicated by the high concentration of urea in the tissue fluids. We found that the most consistent optimum fixation for light microscopic observation was obtained by using an initial fixative consisting of 2% glutaraldehyde–1% paraformaldehyde in a 0.1 M phosphate buffer to which 10% sucrose had been added (Jollie and Jollie, 1967). The final osmolarity, measured cryostatically, was 960–990 mOsm. Following this initial fixation and a buffer rinse, the tissue was postfixed in buffered 1% osmium tetroxide, with all buffers of equivalent osmolarity. The tissue was then dehydrated for embedment in Araldite 502 (Luft, 1961).

Plastic embedments offer several advantages. First, the tissue is suitable for electron microscopic observation, in which case the tissue preservation may be determined by ultrastructural criteria. Second, 0.5- to 0.75-μm sections may be prepared for light microscopic observation. Since 3- to 5-μm-thick sections appear to be the lower limit of sectioning thickness with paraffin embedments, edge contrast will be decreased by the out-of-focus tissue above and below the optical plane. Hence the thinner sections are particularly useful in maximizing contrast. The plastic-embedded tissue must be cut with glass knives on an ultratome using standard electron microscopic sectioning techniques, and toluidine blue may be used to stain the myelinated nerves without the necessity of removing the plastic.

Orientation of the tissue is another important consideration, and begins with the embedding. Since we are interested in measuring cross-sectional dimensions, orientation methods were used to maximize the cross-sectional orientation of the nerve fibers (Brundage and Dunn, 1972*a,b*).

The magnification of the final photographic print requires calibration at two levels; calibration of the light microscope and calibration of the photographic enlarger. A Zeiss Ultraphot equipped with a 40 x planapochromatic oil immersion objective lens was used in taking high-contrast 4- by 5-inch negatives on Kodak Ektapan film. Pictures of a Zeiss standard test specimen were processed with each group of negatives and later served in calibrating the final magnification of the print. Photomicrographs were printed with a point-light source at short exposure times so that maximum development was obtained in 3 min. Attention to the exposure time is important since an overexposed print can result in increased object size (Williams and Wendell-Smith, 1960). Optimally, the final photomicrograph magnification should be 1000 x so that conversion from millimeters to micrometers is direct. However, two additional constraints were placed on the final magnification. First, the photomicrograph should be slightly less than the size of the active area of the tablet used for digitizing; for example, at least one dimension, the Y axis, must fit within this area. Second, the diameter of the smallest fiber must be sufficiently large to be resolved by the operator.

Two final preparatory steps were found useful prior to digitization. First, a bundle contour line should be drawn, on the micrograph, around the nerve bundle at the limits of the epineurium. The contour line aids bundle recognition during display and later serves to estimate the extracellular space within the bundle. Second, each nerve fiber in the bundle should be numbered, a step required in subsequent editing in which the sequence of the operator-guided input must be known.

3. Hardware Requirements

The FORTRAN program system was used with a Digital PDP-11/20 computer having 24 K words of memory and an RK05 disk with a 1.2-million-word capacity. The peripherals included a Tektronix model 4010-1 terminal (keyboard and CRT) and Tektronix 4610 hard-copier. Initially, the graphics input tablet was constructed from a nonfunctioning *X, Y* recorder from which the electronics has been removed. A bias voltage was applied to each of two precision potentiometers whose shafts were mechanically coupled to the position of the stylus along the *X* or *Y* axis. Manual positioning of the stylus resulted in an analog voltage output of the *X* and *Y* axes potentiometers proportional to the position of the stylus. These voltage analogs then served as the input to an analog-to-digital (A/D) converter on the computer system. An interrupt button was also installed on the *X, Y* recorder which initiated the A/D conversion of single events. The active area of this *X, Y* recorder was 7½ by 10 inches in the *X* and *Y* axes, respectively.

Subsequently, the *X, Y* recorder input device was replaced with a GRAF/PEN sonic digitizer, with an active area of 14 by 14 inches, two linear microphones (one for each axis), and a spark-emitting stylus. The time between sound production at the stylus and its detection by the microphones is proportional to the *X, Y* coordinates of the stylus's position and serves as a direct binary input to the PDP-11/20 computer system.

4. The Input Programs

A FORTRAN computer program, FIBER, was written to process the information digitized from the photomicrographs (O'Leary *et al.*, 1976). The A/D, display, and initial edit operations were called from this program as subroutines (Fig. 1). Figure 2 is the flow chart of five PDP-11 assembly language routines, called by FIBER, which control the file manipulation and the A/D sampling.

Fig. 1. Flow chart of the FORTRAN IV program FIBER used in digitizing the nerve bundle contour and the mean diameters of the axon and axon-plus-myelin of nerve bundles. The program also identifies and stores the axon center coordinates, thereby allowing later spatial distribution analyses. The program includes subroutines which permit an oversized bundle (one larger than the active tablet area) to be entered and written as a single file. (From O'Leary *et al.*, 1976.)

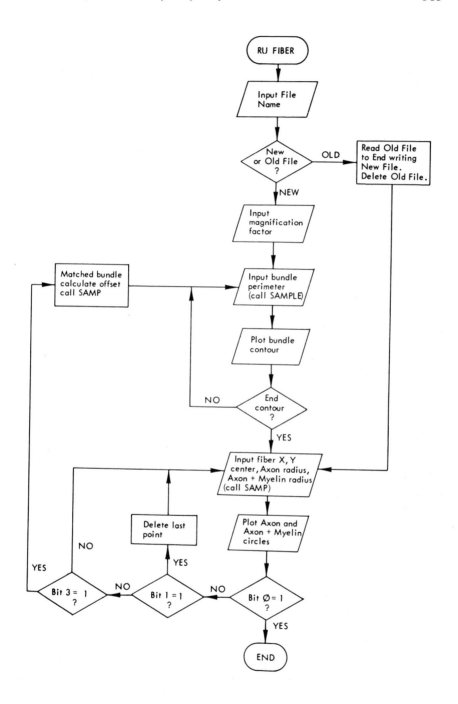

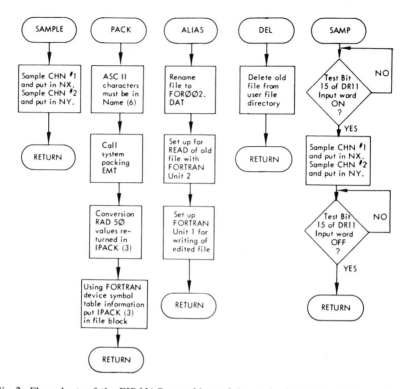

Fig. 2. Flow charts of the FIB.MAC assembly modules, each of which is called by and used with FIBER. SAMPLE is used while entering the bundle contour information and operates as a windowing device for distance-delayed sampling with the distance determined by the operator. PACK condenses nine ASCII characters into three PDP-11 16-bit words and places them into the FORTRAN device table fileblock for unit 1. ALIAS changes the input file name to FOR002.DAT, thereby creating a temporary backup file, and outputs the edited file under the original name. This is used during the initial editing procedures. DEL, when activated, deletes the old file, FOR002.DAT, from the user's file directory, a step which must be completed prior to any additional initial editing operations. SAMP monitors bit 15 of a DR11A 16-bit input word which is activated during fiber digitization by the interrupt button on the graphic input device. The program samples channels 1 and 2 of the ADO 1 A/D converter and places these values in a common block. (From O'Leary *et al.*, 1976.)

The input procedure is summarized as follows:

1. Assign an individual file name.
2. If this is a new file, type in the magnification of the photomicrograph.
3. Input the bundle contour. In this case, the input device is used in a DRAW mode, and the image is displayed on the CRT.
4. Input each fiber's diameters with eight points. In this case, the input device is used as an event marker.
5. Signal the last fiber's entry with bit 1 on the processor switch register.

The assignment of the file name is important since it must contain sufficient information to identify specific individual bundles. The task was simplified because each of our animals were already numbered, each had a right and left side, and we were interested in the horizontal ampullary nerve. Consequently, as an example, the following notation was used:

A352.RH1

The first four characters were the animal number, the next was always a period, the sixth character signified the right (R) or left (L) side, H as the seventh character indicated the horizontal ampullary nerve (HAN), and the final identified the specific nerve bundle (O'Leary *et al.*, 1974). It should be noted that the file (to left of period) contained four characters, while the extension (to the right) contained three. The magnification of the photomicrograph was required in subsequent calculations in which the object size in "tablet units" was converted to image size in micrometers.

As indicated above, the bundle contour information was entered by operating the input device in a DRAW mode. The FIB.MAC subroutine SAMPLE was used to sample the X and Y values from the appropriate channels of the A/D converter, and returned the coordinates to the calling program to be placed in record 1 (Fig. 3). Initially, during the DRAW mode, the stylus positions were automatically sampled and stored sequentially at equal time intervals. The methods of windowing suggested by Cowan and Wann (1973) were used subsequently to advantage. A stationary boundary of 20 tablet units was established around the starting point of the bundle contour, and a boundary of similar dimensions was constructed around the moving stylus. In this double-window sampling technique, the bundle contour was sampled at equal distance intervals. The subroutine continually sampled points until the X, Y values exceeded a minimum distance, at which time the values were stored. This process was repeated, and when the sampled point values were within the value range of the stationary window the program automatically closed the boundary and was ready to accept the individual fiber input data.

Eight points for each individual nerve fiber were entered in the order shown in Fig. 4. The pairs 2,3 and 6,7 were two diameters of the axon corresponding to the inner surface of the myelin sheath. The pairs 1,4 and 5,8 were two diameters of the outer perimeter of the myelin sheath and corresponded to the total fiber dimension, axon plus myelin. It should be remembered that one method used to estimate axon diameters is to optically measure two diameters, average the values, and then record the mean diameters. Mechanically this was accomplished by placing the stylus at each successive point and hitting the interrupt switch. With a minimum of practice, 10−12 sec was required to digitize each fiber and to be ready to input the next. The program FIBER recognized this sequence, 1−8, as the two sets of pairs, 2,3; 6,7 (axon diameters) and 1,4; 5,8 (the axon-plus-myelin diameters). The program

TYPICAL FILE

Record Number 1 Bundle Perimeter Information

1   Number of pairs   Scale factor
2   *X* coordin.   *Y* coordin.
.
.
256

Record Number 2 to *n* (Nerve Fiber Information as 64 Foursomes)

1   *X* Center*   *Y* Center   Axon radius   Axon + myelin radius
5
.
.
.
64

Fig. 3. Details of the file format for FIBER. Record 1, the bundle contour information consists of 512 one-word integers. The first four words contain the number of bundle contour points, the magnification of the photomicrograph, and the center point of the bundle. The subsequent words contain the *X*, *Y* coordinates of points on the bundle perimeter. Record 2 through *n* consists of 256 two-word floating numbers, and contains the *X*, *Y* coordinates of each nerve fiber's center and values in "tablet units" for radii of the axon and axon plus myelin. The *X* position (*) in record 2 indicates several additional situations: a -500 value indicates that the fiber information should be ignored; a -1000 value signals the last fiber in a bundle; and a -2000 value flags the last fiber of a matched or segmented bundle, in which case the program assumes that the following record will contain bundle contour information.

then proceeded to calculate and store the *X*, *Y* coordinates of the center point of the fiber, followed by the mean radii of the axon and axon-plus-myelin which formed record 2 through *n* of the file (Fig. 3). The subroutine SAMP (Fig. 2) was called during this operation. Following the eight-point input, FIBER calculated the circle of best fit based on the mean radii. Points were calculated for all four quadrants by the FIBER subroutine CIRCLE. Results of the calculations were stored as four arrays which were then called out by a PLOT subroutine available to the PDP-11 system. The individual nerve fiber was thus reconstructed and plotted on the CRT as two concentric circles within the bundle contour in the same relative position as on the photomicrograph. This immediate display facilitated rapid verification of the position and relative size of the nerve fiber just entered on the CRT with its counterpart on the photomicrograph (Fig. 5). Two error subroutines were incorporated into FIBER which permitted initial editing while the photomicrograph was still in place on the active tablet.

If an erroneous entry was made prior to entering the eighth, or last, point, bit 1 (bits 0, 1, 2, 3, etc. are switches on the console register) signaled that the temporary buffer was to be zeroed, and the program then accepted entry of the next fiber. If an error was detected after the eighth point had been entered, bit 1 called the subroutine ALIAS (Fig. 2), which first renamed the file and redisplayed the entire bundle contour and nerve fibers minus the last-entered fiber. The new file was renamed to the old file name (Fig. 2).

The process of digitizing the individual nerve fibers was continued until the last fiber of the bundle, which was signaled by setting bit 0 = 1 prior to entering its eight-points. The file was then closed by entering −1000 in the record. Since the majority of the nerve bundles, when printed at a final magnification of 1035x, fitted within the confines of the tablet's active area, no further manipulations were necessary. With several bundles, however, the active area of the tablet proved too small, even at the minimum useful enlargement 810x magnification. Since it was desirable to include all the fibers of bundle in a single logical computer file, it became necessary to digitize discrete segments of the bundle sequentially. This was accomplised by computing an X and Y offset for the second through n segments.

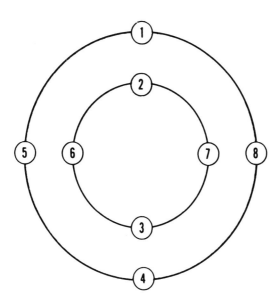

Fig. 4. Schematic of the axon surrounded by a myelin sheath. The numbers indicate the usual position and sequence of the correct input points. While the angle can be rotated, the sequence of input must remain as indicated.

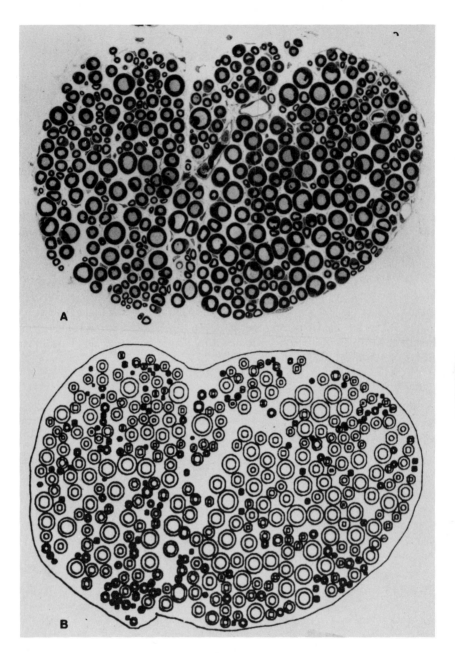

Fig. 5. Comparision of the photomicrograph (A) to the computer display (B). The light micrograph shown in A is a cross-sectioned bundle from the horizontal ampullary nerve of an elasmobranch. The micrograph and computer display have been printed at approximately the same magnification (×280). The immediate display called by FIBER permits rapid verification that all of the fibers were correctly entered.

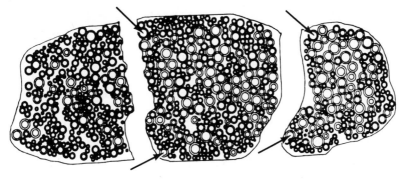

Fig. 6. Computer display of an oversized bundle which is shown as separated segments. The irregular transverse lines are used to enclose areas of the bundle that will fit within the confines of the active tablet area. The two transposition point pairs in each segment (arrows) are utilized to write all of the information in a single file.

The procedure followed for data entry with the X, Y recorder was

1. Align the photomicrograph to the left border of the recorder bed.
2. Enter the data as usual.
3. Set bit 3 = 1 prior to entering the last fiber of the current segment.
4. Input two identifiable points in the next segment.
5. Shift photomicrograph to the left (for increasing X values), to center the next segment and reaffix it to the recorder.
6. Reset bit 3 = 0.
7. Input the same two identifiable points as in step (4).
8. Repeat steps (2)–(7) for each segment.
9. Input the last fiber in the bundle after setting bit 0 = 1.

Oversized bundles required arbitrary segmenting. The boundary contour was drawn followed by transverse lines through the extracellular space so that the segmented areas fit within the active tablet (Fig. 6). File designation and subsequent digitizing followed the stepwise procedure outlined earlier. Setting bit 3 = 1 signaled entry of the last fiber in the segment, which was identified by a value of -2000 in the record. This entry was a signal that the next input would be the offset points followed by contour information. Translocation of oversize bundles was necessary only along the X axis, since at 810x the photomicrographs fit within the Y axis confines of the X, Y recorder. The offset was calculated as the mean difference in X and Y coordinates of the two points in position 2 and position 1. This offset was then added to all X, Y coordinates in subsequent segments, which resulted in values from the entire bundle being stored as a single file. The offsetting procedure could be repeated for any number of segments.

Although the translocation and offset procedure was implemented only in the X axis, identical logic could be used to extend the translocation and offset to the Y axis, thereby allowing large areas in a single plane to be digitized. In effect, it offered the potential to montage adjacent regions digitally as a single file. Moreover, the logic could be extended also into the Z axis, which is perpendicular to the plane of the plotter bed, thereby permitting reconstructions from serial histological sections. In this case, the Z offset value would be the thickness of the sections, which would be only a single value for serial sections of uniform thickness. This single Z value could also be the mean of a range of thicknesses within acceptable limits resulting from variations in thickness from section to section. When thin sectioning for electron microscopy is being considered, this is a necessary and important factor.

The input program FIBER has several advantageous features. First, it allows rapid digitization of fiber information. In addition, it calculates and stores simultaneously the X, Y coordinates of the fiber center and also the mean radii of the axon and axon-plus-myelin as determined from a circle of best-fit calculation. The immediate visual display provides prompt verification and validation of each entry, so that the initial editing steps can be called when needed. Moreover, photomicrographs that are oversized in the X dimension can be digitized and stored as a single file.

5. The Editing Programs

Prior to the final analysis, it was necessary to compare the stored information with the original photomicrograph for accuracy, for example, to ensure that each fiber had been properly entered and that no erroneous entries were made while digitizing (Dunn *et al.*, 1975). The program FIBDIS enabled the operator to recall and display any given bundle of nerves for the purpose of verification, and to complete this operation without reopening the file (Fig. 7).

The errors most frequently encountered were (1) failure to enter one or more fibers, (2) erroneous entries such as double entry or improper dimensions, and (3) improper entry of the magnification which resulted from typing the wrong character. These errors were detected usually after the photomicrograph had been removed from the active tablet, and hence editing capabilities were required in addition to those available in FIBER. The program FIBOUT was designed to serve two functions: display of the recorded information and editing (Fig. 8). The WRITE OUT function was useful in verifying such factors as complete bundle entry and inclusion of the magnification. The EDIT portion served to rectify the common errors mentioned above.

The "D" option in FIBOUT allowed either the magnification to be changed or fibers to be deleted. The "D" decision initiated a terminal listing of

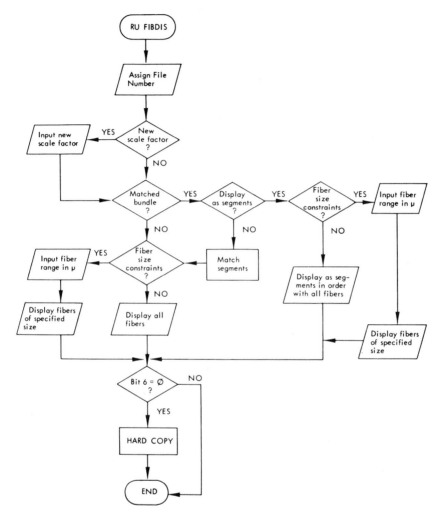

Fig. 7. Flow chart of the FORTRAN IV program FIBDIS, which allows the bundle to be displayed either as a complete bundle or in segmented form and either with all fibers included or with specified fiber size constraints.

the boundary contour file to the end, after which the magnification could be changed or not as required. Thereupon the fiber files were printed record by record. Following each record, the operator had the option of editing as many fibers as necessary. The editing involved deleting a fiber by substituting −500 in the X position as an indicator to ignore that fiber. The insertion of missed fibers, activated by the "I" option of FIBOUT, was more involved than simple fiber

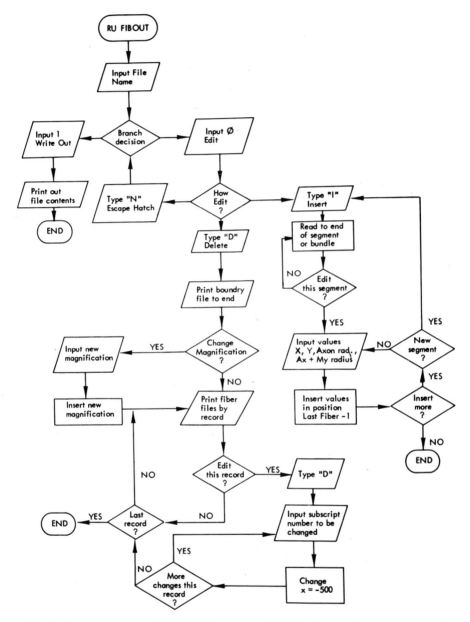

Fig. 8. Flow chart of the FORTRAN IV program FIBOUT, allowing the operator to read the file contents or edit the data. The editing portion of the program consists of four subroutines: "N" serves as a direct escape route in case the edit portion was erroneously called; "I" permits input of fibers which either have been omitted or are in need of change; "D" deletes specified fibers in case of erroneous entry; and "C" allows the magnification to be corrected.

deletion. The FIBOUT "I" option required prior determination of the X, Y coordinates and the axon and axon-plus-myelin radii values. The appropriate X and Y coordinates could generally be determined directly from neighboring axons. For example, the Y coordinate could be determined by placing a straight edge (a navigator's parallel ruler) through the center of the fiber, and parallel to the X axis. The edge was then traced to locate a nearby fiber whose Y center coordinate was identical to that of the fiber being inserted. A similar process was completed for the X coordinate. The two radii were determined as follows:

1. Attach the micrograph to the graphic input recorder's active surface.
2. Open a temporary test file in FIBER, i.e., TEST.RH1.
3. Repeat the eight-point input process for the fiber to be inserted (enter with bit 1 = 1).
4. Read the radii from the FIBOUT writeout option.
5. Delete the test file from the user's directory.

Once the four values were determined, the "I" option in the FIBOUT edit option read to the end of the segment or bundle. The new values were then entered via the teletype terminal keyboard and inserted in the position preceding the -1000. This step procedure could be repeated as often as necessary.

6. The Analysis Programs

The numerical information was derived from the program FIBHST (Fig. 9), which computed or plotted the following information for either axon or axon-plus-myelin: mean diameter in micrometers (M), standard deviation (SD), coefficient of variation (CV = SD/M), the number of fibers, the maximum and minimum diameters, plots of the number of fibers by diameter increments (operator determined) in histogram form, and finally displays of the bin contents (Fig. 10). This information could be calculated by individual bundles or by batch processing for multiple bundles (e.g., right side vs. left side, animal vs. animal, entire sample group). As another option, a scattergram of the myelin thickness was computed and displayed as a function of axon diameter. Again the same batch-processing capabilities were possible as with the histograms. The computed scattergrams permitted further the opportunity for curve fitting to define precisely the relationship between myelin thickness and axon diameter. Additional numerical relationships could easily be incorporated such as plots of myelin thickness vs. number, ratios of myelin thickness to axon diameter plotted vs. percent, and the reconstruction of the compound action potential (Landau *et al.*, 1968; Tapp, 1974).

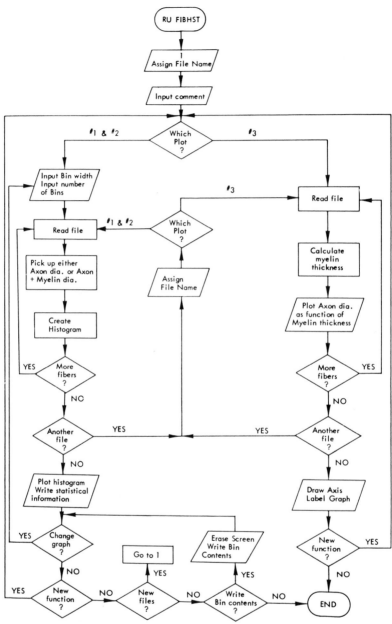

Fig. 9. Flow chart of FIBHST, a FORTRAN IV program used in analysis of the data. Three subroutines currently comprise this program: #1 calls out a display of the axon diameter in histogram form with the statistics shown to the right in Fig. 9; #2 displays the histogram and statistics of the axon plus myelin; and #3 calls a plot where the axon diameter is expressed as a function of myelin thickness. This program also permits batch processing as well as single-bundle-analysis capabilities.

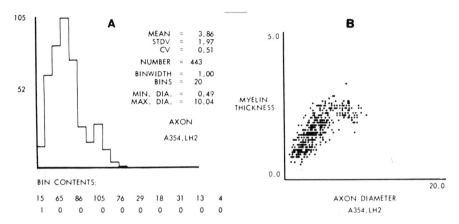

Fig. 10. An axon diameter histogram (A) and a myelin thickness–axon diameter plot (B) as called from FIBHST. Both statistical and numerical information characterizing the callout is shown to the right of the histogram. Prior to the histogram display, the operator must designate the bin width (in Micrometers) and the number of bins. After the display, several operator options remain: the bin widths and/or the number of bins may be changed without reentering the programs; the bin contents may be called (shown here below the histogram); the axon-plus-myelin and the myelin thickness–axon diameter plot may be called without further assignment; or the program may be terminated.

The program FIBHST began with a DIMENSION statement, which allowed forming a tabulated array of the nerve fiber data stored by FIBER. Since the original data file consisted of four columns (the X coordinate, the Y coordinate, the axon radius, and the axon-plus-myelin radius) and each row contained this information on a single nerve fiber, the analysis array was easily formed by beginning, for example, with the axon radius of the first fiber and incrementing each subsequent entry to the analysis array by 4. Batch processing then simply extended the analysis array from 1 to n files as specified by the operator.

As mentioned earlier, the program FIBDIS called up a graphic display of any given bundle. Not only could the entire fiber be displayed, but fiber size constraints could be superimposed on the display. For example, specific fiber size ranges could be called for display to the exclusion of all others. Figure 11 is an example of the results of this sieving technique in which the fibers have been displayed in 4-μm increments. This type of display permits the spatial distribution of nerve fiber size groups to be readily recognized, and it retains a wide variability in the size constraints which the operator can determine.

Another method used to provide information concerning spatial distribution involves an analysis of fiber size distribution by bundle area. One technique

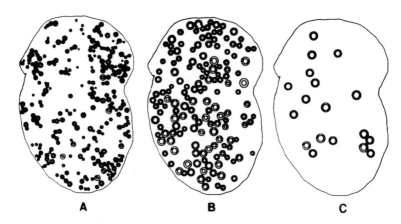

Fig. 11. An example of a bundle display with size constraints on the axon diameter. This is the same bundle as displayed in Fig. 5 but with the following size constraints which were operator determined: (A) 0–3.99 μm, (B) 4.00–7.99 μm, and (C) 8–12 μm. This variable-sieving technique is a useful procedure to determine and depict obvious size distributions of fibers within a bundle.

requires that the nerve bundle be divided into regions of equal area. Donovan (1967) used this approach to analyze the optic nerve by constructing radials at 30° intervals and then forming concentric circles such that all regions had equal areas regardless of their shape. We have adopted a spiderweb matrix approach in which eight radials at 45° intervals were constructed from the center of the bundle to its periphery. Each of the radials was then bisected and a line was constructed joining each radial's center point. The advantages of a spiderweb matrix over an equal-area matrix was that the former was geometrically very simple and straightforward to construct initially, and the number of regions could be increased simply by bisecting further each segment of the radial. Additionally, the segment areas could be made more equal simply by using a point 0.70 along the radial from the origin rather than bisecting. Individual regions were identified by number, such that the odd numbers corresponded to the peripheral regions and even numbers to the central. The computations of interest would require the following information from each region: the number of nerve fibers per region and the mean, standard deviation, and coefficient of variation of the axon diameters, the overall fiber diameters, and the area of the region. These parameters would permit the fiber density to be calculated as well as the spatial distribution by size throughout the bundle of nerve fibers. The coordinates of the fiber center would assign the fiber within or on the boundary of a specific region.

7. Discussion

The uniqueness of the system presented here lies in the application of computer graphics to the measurement of axon and nerve fiber dimensions and the eight-point algorithm used to digitize these measurements. The advantages are several, and they relate primarily to the rapidity of input, which allows sampling of a large population in a relatively short time and the analysis of many parameters from a single direct input, as well as expansion of the analysis at a later time.

Our basic approach has been to maintain a maximum operator–computer interactive input relationship. Several techniques are available whereby the information contained pictorially in the photomicrograph may be digitized automatically or semiautomatically (Hildebrand, quoted by Hall and Ronning-Arnesen, 1974; Llinás and Hillman, 1975; Reddy *et al.*, 1973; Selverston, 1973; Ware and LoPresti, 1975), methods which could easily be applied when dealing with essentially two contrast levels obtained in the toluidine blue-stained sections of myelinated nerves in this study. However, when the number of contrast levels, the gray levels, is increased considerably, the demand for programming recognition results in greatly increased computer capacity requirements. Further, digitization of all information contained in the micrograph is not always required, a task that can quickly exhaust the memory capabilities of the computer. Hence, by retaining the operator-decision feature, not only is the small computer sufficient but also the maximum in flexibility is retained.

The classical methods of manually measuring the mean diameters of nerve fibers are very time consuming. For example, approximately 110 man-hr was required to measure the fiber diameters of a single horizontal ampullary nerve consisting of approximately 1400 fibers. Results from the manual measurements must be calculated from typed data, which requires additional time, is a potential source of error, and provides no information concerning spatial distribution. A total of approximately 86 man-hr was required with the computer graphics system to input fibers comprising the horizontal ampullary nerves from both sides of six animals for a total in excess of 17,000 nerve fibers.

The process of calculating the mean diameter from two diameters is certainly a well-established anatomical technique. There are, however, many potential sources of error. One such error is due to volume changes in the tissue caused during dehydration and embedding of the sample (Williams and Wendell-Smith, 1960; Romero and Skoglund, 1965). Estimates of as much as a 10% volume change have been reported (Donovan, 1967) using plastic-embedded nervous tissue and even more in muscle tissue (Eisenberg and Mobley, 1975). Another error resulting from improper tissue orientation is elliptically shaped rather than circular nerve profiles, an error easily recognized visually and corrected by repositioning and resectioning of the block. In the vicinity of the Schwann cell nucleus, the axon generally becomes flattened on one side; however, it is usually possible to choose the diameters at directions which will minimize the effect of flattening upon the diameter. Variations in the myelin perimeters produce another series of potential errors, and they generally involve only the internal perimeter, which obviously affects the axon diameter measurements. Some instances in which the internal surface is crenulated have been reported (Berthold and Carlstedt, 1973), but were encountered only very infrequently in the present study. Another alteration of the myelin appears in the light microscope as a separation located within the myelin sheath, resulting in a multilamellar appearance. These regions may or may not represent Schmidt–Lanterman clefts. One method by which this "error" could be corrected would be to determine a mean number of myelin membranes per unit distance. Then the true myelin thickness in those fibers showing separations could easily be determined by counting the number of myelin membranes. This latter appraoch would entail observations on an electron microscopic level, in which case the percentage of fibers exhibiting the separations should determine whether or not these corrections are necessary.

The eight-point input algorithm is required in our study since we are working essentially with a rod (the axon) within a tube (the myelin sheath), and are interested in the diameters of both. Broader applicability of this program system could be accomplished simply by changing from an eight-point to a four-point input requirement. The system could then be applied directly to measuring mean diameters of subcellular particles as mitochondria or synaptic vesicles (Dunn *et al.*, 1968; Peter *et al.*, 1970) or to cellular profiles, e.g., cross-sectional dimensions of the outer segments of visual cells (Dunn, 1969). With further modification to a two-point algorithm, this same system could permit measurement of membrane dimensions, allowing rapid sampling of these linear dimensions.

This is then a system which allows acquisition of numerical information with retention of the spatial distribution of that information, all based on a single direct input from cross-sections of individual nerve fibers. Further, the rapidity of the input permits a statistically significant sampling within a reasonable length of time.

ACKNOWLEDGMENTS

This investigation was supported by NIH Research Grants NS-09440, NS-09692, and NS-09823 from the National Institute of Neurological and Communicative Disorders and Stroke.

8. References

Berthold, C.-H., and Carlstedt, T., 1973, Fixation and numerical estimation of myelinated nerve fibres during initial myelination in the cat, *Neurobiology* 3:1–18.

Bohman, S.-O., 1974, The ultrastructure of the rat renal medulla as observed after improved fixation methods, *J. Ultrastruct. Res.* 47:329–360.

Brundage, M. J., and Dunn, R. F., 1972a, Flat end embedding and re-embedding of specimens, *J. Ultrastruct. Res.* 38:222.

Brundage, M. J., and Dunn, R. F., 1972b, Re-embedding of specimens for maximum orientation, in: *Electron Microscopy 1972* (C. J. Arceneaux, ed.), pp. 696–697, Claitor's Publ. Div., Baton Rouge.

Cowan, W. M., and Wann, D. F., 1973, A computer system for the measurement of cell and nuclear sizes, *J. Microsc.* 99:331–348.

Donovan, A., 1967, The nerve fibre composition of the cat optic nerve, *J. Anat.* 101:1–11.

Dunn, R. F., 1969, The dimensions of rod outer segments related to light absorption in the gecko retina, *Vision Res.* 9:603–609.

Dunn, R. F., Worsfold, M., and Peter, J. B., 1968, The morphology and biochemistry of isolated skeletal muscle mitochondria, in: *Electron Microscopy 1968* (C. J. Arceneaux, ed.), p. 124, Claitor's Pub. Div., Baton Rouge.

Dunn, R. F., O'Leary, D. P., and Kumley, W. E., 1975, Quantitative analysis of micrographs by computer graphics, *J. Microsc.* 105:205–213.

Eisenberg, B. R., and Mobley, B. A., 1975, Size changes in single muscle fibers during fixation and embedding, *Tissue Cell* 7:383–387.

Eisenberg, B. R., Kuda, A. M., and Peter, J. B., 1974, Stereological analysis of mammalian skeletal muscle, *J. Cell Biol.* 60:732–754.

Fernand, V. S., and Young, J. Z., 1951, The sizes of the nerve fibres of muscle cells, *Proc. Royal Soc. London Ser. B* 139:38–58.

Hall, J. G., and Rønning-Arnesen, A., 1974, An electron-microscopical analysis of the square areas and diameters of the cochlear nerve fibers in cats, *Acta Otolaryngol.* 77:305–310.

Jollie, W. P., and Jollie, L. G., 1967, Electron microscopic observations on the yolk sac of the spiny dogfish, *Squalus acanthis, J. Ultrastruct. Res.* 18:102–126.

Karlsson, U., and Schultz, R. L., 1965, Fixation of the central nervous system for electron microscopy by aldehyde perfusion, *J. Ultrastruct. Res.* 12:160–186.

Landau, W. M., Clare, M. H., and Bishop, G. H., 1968, Reconstruction of myelinated nerve tract action potentials: An arithmetic method, *Exp. Neurol.* 22:480–490.

Llinás, R., and Hillman, D. E., 1975, A multipurpose tridimensional reconstruction computer system for neuroanatomy, in: *Perspectives in Neurobiology* (M. Santini, ed.), pp. 71–79, Raven Press, New York.

Luft, J. H., 1961, Improvements in epoxy resin embedding methods, *J. Biophys. Biochem. Cytol.* 9:409–414.

Matthews, M. A., 1968, An electron microscopic study of the relationship between axon diameter and initiation of myelin production in the peripheral nervous system, *Anat. Rec.* 161:337–352.

Matthews, M. A., and Duncan, D., 1971, A quantitative study of morphological changes accompanying the initiation and progress of myelin production in the dorsal funiculus of the rat spinal cord, *J. Comp. Neurol.* 142:1–22.

O'Leary, D. P., Dunn, R. F., and Honrubia, V., 1974, Functional and anatomical correlation of afferent responses from the isolated semicircular canal, *Nature (London)* 251:225–227.

O'Leary, D. P., Dunn, R. F., and Kumley, W. E., 1976, On-line computerized entry and display of nerve fiber cross-sections using single or segmented histological records, *Comp. Biomed. Res.* 9:229–237.

Peter, J. B., Fiehn, W., and Dunn, R. F., 1970, Biochemistry and morphology of fragmented sarcoplasmic reticulum, in: *Electron Microscopy 1970* (C. J. Arceneaux, ed.), p. 90, Claitor's Pub. Div., Baton Rouge.

Reddy, D. R., Davis, W., Ohlander, R., and Bihary, D., 1973, Computer analysis of neuronal structure, in: *Intracellular Staining in Neurobiology* (S. B. Kater and C. Nicholson, eds.), pp. 227–253, Springer-Verlag, New York.

Romero, C., and Skoglund, S., 1965, Methodological studies of the technique in measuring nerve fibre diameters, *Acta Morphol. Neerl.-Scand.* 6:107–114.

Selverston, A. J., 1973, The use of intracellular dye injections in the study of small neural networks, in: *Intracellular Staining in Neurobiology* (S. B. Kater, and C. Nicholson, eds.), pp. 255–280, Springer-Verlag, New York.

Sjöstrand, F. S., 1967, *Electron Microscopy of Cells and Tissues*, Vol. 1, Academic Press, New York.

Tapp, R. L., 1974, Axon numbers and distribution myelin thickness, and the reconstruction of the compound action potential in the optic nerve of the teleost: *Eugerres plumieri, J. Comp. Neurol.* 153:267–274.

Ware, R. W., and LoPresti, V., 1975, Three dimensional reconstructions from serial sections, *Int. Rev. Cytol.* 40:325–440.

Weibel, E. R., 1973, Stereological techniques for electron microscopic morphometry, in: *Principles and Techniques of Electron Microscopy*, Vol. 3 (M. A. Hayat, ed.), pp. 237–296, Van Nostrand Reinhold, New York.

Williams, P. L., and Wendell-Smith, C. P., 1960, The use of fixed and stained sections in quantitative studies of peripheral nerve, *Q. J. Microsc. Sci.* 101:43–54.

7

A Computer-Controlled Microscope as a Device for Evaluating Autoradiographs

P. J. R. Boyle and D. G. Whitlock

1. Introduction

In this chapter, we will describe the application of a computer-controlled microscope to the quantitative evaluation of tissue autoradiographs. In our laboratory, we interfaced a microscope to a PDP-12 computer in 1972. Since that time, the system has been applied to various aspects of autoradiographic evaluation of nerves labeled with tritiated amino acids. Similar devices are now available commercially (Altman, 1963; Prensky, 1971), and several have been described in the literature (Boyle and Whitlock, 1974; Stengel-Rutkowski et al., 1974; Wann et al., 1974). Computers have been used with microscopes in other applications for some time (Garvey et al., 1972, 1973; Glaser and Van der Loos, 1965; Izzo and Coles, 1962; Ledley, 1964).

The evaluation of autoradiographs by traditional manual means is time consuming and tedious. Manual methods are also notoriously unreliable (Rodgers, 1973). For these reasons, the development of an automatic means for evaluating autoradiographs has been attempted, over the years, with a wide variety of very ingenious devices (Dendy, 1960; Dudley and Pelc, 1953; Gullberg, 1959; Mazia et al., 1955; Tolles, 1959). However, of these devices only two have received any degree of general acceptance, namely the photometric and computer—microscope methods. Both of these methods have features which limit their application to suitable material. Hence the general objective of a device that will quantitatively evaluate any autoradiograph automatically has not yet been attained. Nevertheless, much progress has been made and computer-controlled microscopes can substantially improve the accuracy and convenience of autoradiograph evaluations.

P. J. R. Boyle and D. G. Whitlock · Department of Anatomy, University of Colorado Medical Center, Denver, Colorado 80220.

2. Material

We label neuronal pathways by injecting certain nerve cell body populations with tritiated amino acids. The tissue containing the processes into which this label is carried is removed from the animal after an appropriate postinjection survival time and is prepared by standard autoradiographic techniques similar to those described by Kopriwa and Le Blond (1962). The tissue is fixed, embedded in paraffin, and sectioned. Ribbons of such sections are placed on microscope slides and dipped in Kodak NTB-2 emulsion. The dipped slides are placed in a cool, dark environment for several weeks, during which time the radiochemical exposes the emulsion. Finally, the exposed silver halide crystals in the emulsion are developed using Kodak D-19.

In these autoradiographs, the position and density of the silver grains indicate the location and, to a degree, the quantity of tritium label in the underlying tissue. This information may be useful in the following forms: The label may be distributed selectively over portions of a relatively large specimen, such as a spinal cord section. In this case, the investigator would seek to know which areas of the specimen are significantly more labeled than others. There may also be a selective labeling of tissue features, for example, some nerve axons may be labeled and others not. In this case, the investigator may wish to distinguish significantly labeled features from other adjacent tissue elements. He may also require a count of these labeled structures or a calculation of the percentage of them present in a specific area of tissue.

Our device has been programmed in ways directed to the accomplishment of the goals outlined above.

3. Hardware

We use a PDP-12A computer (Fig. 1) for a variety of purposes including the tasks described here. It has a disk drive and 32K of memory. Most of the mainframe options have been implemented and have been found useful in autoradiograph evaluation. These options include a point-plot cathode-ray tube, a programmable clock, eight analog input channels, and an extended arithmetic element. The floating-point processor and priority interrupt options have not been implemented.

The microscope (Fig. 2) is a Zeiss Universal with optical paths to the eyepiece, a 35-mm camera, and a television camera. The cameras are connected to the microscope using a Zeiss-supplied head intended for a photometer and a custom-machined fitting. This method of mounting results in a field of view for the television camera which is about 1/35 of the area visible at the eyepiece.

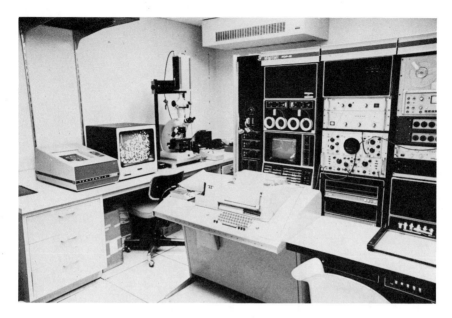

Fig. 1. The PDP-12 and microscope arrangement.

A Zeiss-supplied motorized stage is used. It can be positioned anywhere in a 25- by 75-mm area either manually or under computer control. The light source is a 100-W quartz halogen lamp driven by a programmable D.C. power supply to assure stable intensity.

Another Zeiss-supplied device is a box which contains a two-axis joy stick used to direct the movement of the stage. This movement is programmed in multiples of one $0.5\,\mu$m or in multiples of the field of view of the television camera.

The television camera is conventional and uses the American standard scan and interlace. Because the illumination is limited, a Plumbicon tube is used. It was selected to have no black defects and only very minor white defects. The selection of the Plumbicon was also determined by the need for a tube with even response over the image area, a suitable spectral response, and low image retention even after an extended period of viewing the same field.

The analog video signal from the television camera is fed to a contrast-enhancing amplifier (Fig. 3). Using contrast enhancement to modify the analog signal prior to digitization allows the 64 levels that the analog-to-digital converter can deliver to span only that region of the gray scale which is of primary interest in the particular application. This device operates by removing the synchronizing pulses from the video signal, amplifying the result, adding an

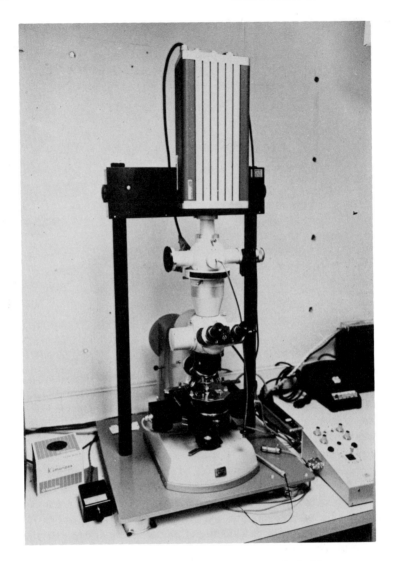

Fig. 2. The microscope with motor-driven controls and television camera.

offset voltage, and reintroducing the synchronizing pulses. Commercial devices which perform this function are available.

After the contrast enhancement, the video signal is converted to a slow-scan form by a bandwidth compressor and digitized into six bits for each of 512 x 512 image points. Then 256 data points are taken from the first or second

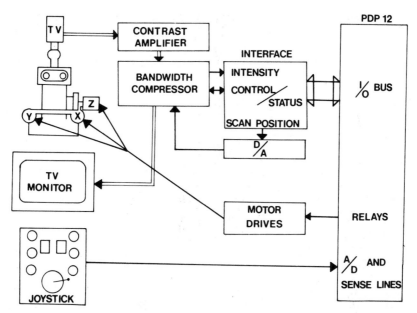

Fig. 3. System block diagram.

interlace under computer control and buffered in a 256 × 6 bit memory. The digital information is then read out by the computer one value at a time.

The data values correspond to the intensities at a preset distance from the left of the frame for each of the scan lines in the raster. Thus one array of 256 points contains the intensities along a vertical line of the image. Since there are two interlaces, a total of 512 intensities are available at each horizontal position.

The acquisition time for a single image with a bandwidth compressor is about 17 sec, which is much slower than that of some more complex devices.

The bandwidth compressor inserts an overlay display on the video signal before it is sent to a television monitor. On the monitor can be seen the original or contrast-enhanced image as well as the digital information being made available to the computer. The resulting composite display is essential for initial adjustment of the analog devices in the processing chain. These displays are shown in Fig. 4. Figure 4A shows the normal television image. The position from which a scan column is being taken is indicated by the line at the arrow, and the brightness along this line is shown by the waveform on the left of the screen. Figure 4B shows the effect of contrast enhancement. The brightness waveform can be seen to have a greater amplitude.

In addition to microscope-related devices, we have used a Tektronix 4014 storage display terminal to provide graphic output which is helpful in visualizing the results of the processing of the television image.

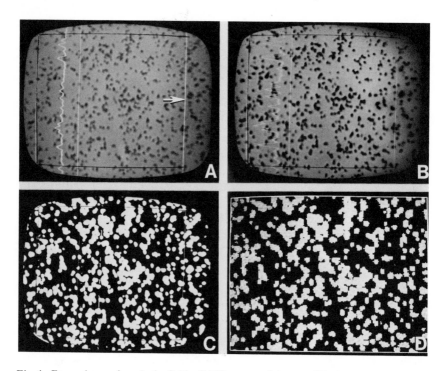

Fig. 4. Four views of a single field. (A) The normal image. (B) The contrast-enhanced image. (C) The dark-field image. (D) The binary image.

A video hard-copy unit has been used to provide a permanent record of the progress of a scan composed of many individual frames. The paper picture that the hard-copy unit produces can also be digitized with a spark-pen tablet if other geometrical properties are to be evaluated.

In the future, we will include a scan converter in the system in order to allow direct annotation of the video monitor image. This addition will provide a means of indexing the frames by their position relative to the specimen as a whole. It will also be helpful in evaluating the process of the more complex frame-processing algorithms since the results can be directly overlaid on the original picture.

4. Principles

Traditionally, the density of silver on an autoradiograph has been determined by manually counting the number of apparent silver grains under a light microscope. This count is taken as a measure of the degree of exposure of the emulsion to the radiochemical and hence as an indicator of the amount of radioactively labeled tracer isotope in the underlying tissue. Grain counts are only one possible measure of exposure. However, when the evaluation must be made manually there does not appear to be any alternative to grain counting.

While grain counting is very reasonable at the electron microscopic level with the special emulsions and procedures that can be used in that case, it is somewhat questionable at the light level. This difficulty arises because the emulsions used for light autoradiographs, as well as the development and exposure times, must be selected to produce silver which is visible under light. These procedures result in a distribution of silver not clearly related to the number of silver halide crystals which were actually exposed by the radiochemical. An example of such a difficulty is illustrated in Fig. 5A, which is an electron micrograph of an autoradiograph prepared for light as described above. In this example, it is not at all clear how many silver halide crystals were involved. Because of this ambiguity, measures of exposure other than grain counts are desirable. The optical density of a developed photographic emulsion is known to be linearly related to the exposure over a wide range (Altman,

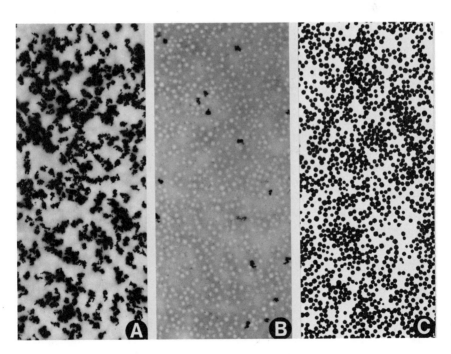

Fig. 5. Three electron micrographs of NTB-2 emulsion. (A) 1:1 dilution, developed. (B) 1:4 dilution, developed. (C) Undeveloped.

1963). Therefore, the area of the specimen obscured by silver is one reasonable measure of exposure. Devices which use area as the measured quantity have been described a number of times (Mazia *et al.*, 1955; Stengel-Rutkowski *et al.*, 1974), but the area property has not been carefully studied. Mertz (1969) did present some area distribution results, but the fact that area measures are a function of the lighting and optics used makes these results rather limited.

Area measurements have the advantage that they are easily and reliably determined by a computer-controlled microscope. In applications where area measures are determined by our device, we have found results similar to those reported by Stengel-Rutkowski *et al.* (1974), namely, that area measures are, on the average, proportional to the visual counts at low-to-medium densities.. This result is to be expected since the silver halide crystals in NTB-2 emulsion are remarkably uniform in size. Figure 5C is an electron micrograph of an undeveloped NTB-2 emulsion in which the crystal uniformity is apparent.

In light autoradiographs, the emulsion is usually not a monolayer. The developed silver has a three-dimensional distribution. Therefore, at the higher silver densities a measure which is affected by the surface area of the silver rather than its projected area will be more responsive. This argument favors incident light (dark-field) photometry. Photometry is a well-documented means for evaluating the level of exposure of autoradiographs. The arguments in its favor were presented as early as 1959 (Gullberg, 1959), and it has been compared favorably to manual methods by many authors since then (Dendy, 1960; Rodgers, 1961, 1962). A computer-controlled microscope can perform a photometric function well while providing a high degree of control over the area being measured and without the errors introduced by diaphragms because of the Swartzchild–Villiger effect (Howling and Fitzgerald, 1959).

There are cases in which it is desirable to count the number of silver "blobs" over an area of the specimen. Very low densities of silver in a highly dilute emulsion represent one such case. Figure 5B is an electron micrograph of a partially exposed NTB-2 emulsion diluted 1:4. Here the silver halide crystals are separated and the developed silver arising from individual crystals has a high probability of being distinct. Thus it is reasonable to assume a correspondence between the number of silver blobs and the degree of exposure of the emulsion to the radiochemical, and hence to use blob counts as a measure of exposure. Another case in which blobs must be counted occurs when very dense aggregates of developed silver appear over certain labeled features of the specimen and a count of these features is required. In this case, the number of such features corresponds to the number of distinguishable silver aggregates. Figure 6 is an example of such a case. Here heavily labeled axons in a nerve have produced dense silver aggregates. These axons are to be counted rather than individually evaluated. Counting the number of separate objects in the field of view is another of the operations which a computer-controlled microscope performs easily

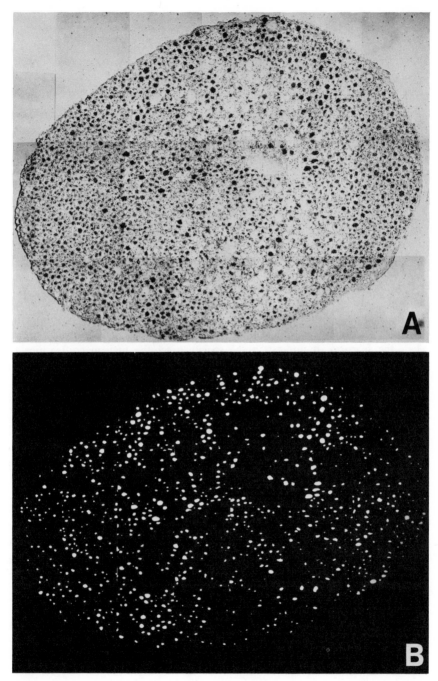

Fig. 6. Cross-section of a nerve with labeled axons. (A) The transmitted light image. (B) The processed binary result.

There are cases in which completely automatic evaluation of the autoradiograph is not practical. As computer programs become more sophisticated, there are fewer of these cases but at present it is still necessary to have some programs available which rely on the investigator to distinguish the features that he wishes to evaluate.

5. Software

A computer-controlled microscope has two separately automated parts: the stage movement and the TV picture digitizer. The algorithms applied to these two parts are distinct so that a given program which scans a specimen in a selected way can be coupled with a variety of different algorithms for processing the picture at each frame of the scan.

5.1. Stage Control

A stepping-motor-driven stage provides the ability to position the specimen accurately on a coordinate system. This facility becomes most useful when the features of interest in the specimen require high magnifications to make them visible. When high magnifications are used, only a small portion of the specimen is in view at any one time. Thus the relative positions of parts of the specimen are difficult to visualize and a systematic scan of a large area is simply not possible manually.

The first thing that a motor-driven stage can make possible is a program which allows the investigator to construct a map of his specimen referenced to a coordinate system (Fig. 7). He can, for example, scan around the edges of the tissue and have an outline of the tissue drawn on a plotter. He can then find reference features in the specimen and have them marked by the plotter. Since these points are on the same coordinate system, the resultant data can be used to measure sizes and distances as well as help visualize later data. One use of this facility in our laboratory has been to obtain size measurements of axons in spinal cord cross-sections. Other investigators have used similar devices to trace Golgi-impregnated neurons (Wann *et al.*, 1973) and for general distance measurement (Shinn amd Kline, 1968).

Once the specimen has been mapped, it is a simple matter to program a systematic scan of it, successively bringing adjacent frames into view. In each frame, silver grains or other features of interest can be quantified.

In some cases, it is adequate to evaluate only parts of the specimen. Suitable programming can leave the investigator free to position the viewing frame anywhere and the resultant data can still be added to the specimen map in the correct position.

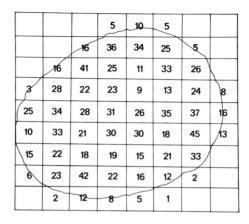

Fig. 7. Tissue map with the axon counts from the cross-section in Fig. 6.

5.2. Frame Processing

As mentioned earlier, it will always be necessary to use the investigator in some frame-processing tasks. Thus the first step in frame processing is to provide a means of input that allows the investigator to communicate with the computer conveniently. In addition to the array of buttons, knobs, and the joy stick used for stage control, we have a simple felt-tipped pen with a microswitch attached to it which we have found most useful. The switch makes it possible for the computer to determine whether the pen point is in contact with the TV monitor screen (Fig. 8). The investigator can use this pen to mark, on the monitor, the objects he wishes to count. Then the computer merely counts the number of surface contacts of the pen. In this way, counts of unlabeled or ambiguous objects can be made without the fatigue or duplication associated with traditional methods.

If the frame is an autoradiograph viewed under incident light adjusted to illuminate the emulsion layer, then two automatic measures of exposure are easily computed. The first is the proportion of the frame covered by developed silver in the emulsion. This is computed by simply counting the number of image points where the light intensity exceeds a fixed level. The second is the total amount of light reflected by the developed silver. This is computed by summing the digitized intensity over all the image points.

These measures are repeatable to 1%. Manual evaluations (Lajtha *et al.*, 1958), photometric devices (Dendy, 1960), and devices which count individual grains by transmitted light (Wann *et al.*, 1974) typically give about 10% repeatability. The use of dark-field illumination reduces the effects of tissue and stain variations and produces a very high-contrast image. Simple functions of

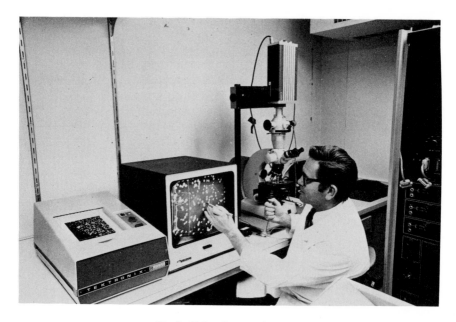

Fig. 8. Using the counting pen.

low-noise dark-field images, such as the area or integral measures, are very stable. Our experience indicates that similar functions of transmitted light images require more complex noise-removal processing in order to produce sound results.

Both area and integral measures of exposure are affected by the optical settings of the microscope. In particular, the magnification used determines the size of the area of the specimen that corresponds to each image point. To make the measurements more universal, we divide them by the average value obtained for a visually isolated silver grain under the same conditions.

Blob counting is slightly more complex, but, provided that the blobs are solid masses which contrast with the tissue background, the task is still quite simple. In our device, the contrast-enhancing amplifier can be used to create this massed effect in many cases where the unmodified image would not have sufficient contrast. Analog or digital low-pass filtering of the video signal can also be helpful here.

The first task in blob counting is to obtain a clear binary image. This means that the gray tones of the original image must be separated into light and dark in such a way that the resultant image does not have isolated light points in the dark areas or *vice versa*. With silver under incident lighting a suitable image can be obtained by applying a simple threshold to the digitized intensity and then correcting the isolated errors, i.e., the so-called salt-and-pepper noise.

The number of solid separate blobs in the resultant picture is given by a simple topological property called its Euler number. This quantity can be computed by counting (1) the number of light points L, (2) the number of pairs of adjacent light points P, and (3) the number of foursomes of adjacent light points F. Then the number of blobs is $N = L + F - P$. This number reflects the number of blobs if the blobs do not have holes and if diagonal connectedness is not required (Fig. 9). A comprehensive discussion of the Euler number property has been presented by Duda and Hart (1973).

In cases where incident lighting does not apply, such as when objects differentiated by the tissue stain are being distinguished, the problem of obtaining a suitable binary image is more complicated. Edge-extraction algorithms are usually necessary. While there exist some very effective edge-extraction algorithms such as that described by Hueckel (1971, 1973), these generally consume too much computer time to be practical for real-time applications. Differentiating edge extractors offer a compromise which is frequently effective. A discussion of this type of image processing is beyond the scope of this chapter, but a full presentation is given by Rosenfeld (1969; Rosenfeld and Thurston, 1971). We have applied differentiators satisfactorily to medium-contrast images (Boyle and Whitlock, 1974). At this point, the limits of the device are being approached and the degree of success achieved will vary with the particular specimen used and the skill of the operator in setting the processing parameters.

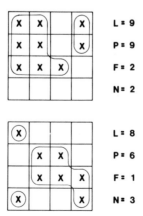

Fig. 9. Euler number computations, illustrating that diagonal connectedness is not used.

6. *Conclusion*

A computer-controlled microscope provides a general tool with a wide range of applications. It makes the task of interpreting autoradiographs less tedious and more exact than with the traditional methods. In addition, since it is a software-oriented device it can be modified to take advantage of new techniques as they become available, as well as perform other unrelated tasks at other times.

ACKNOWLEDGMENTS

This research was supported, in part, by NIH Grants NS-08453-06 and NS-08009-06.

7. *References*

Altman, J., 1963, Regional ultilization of leucine-^{3}H by normal rat brain: Microdensito-metric evaluation of autoradiographs, *J. Histochem. Cytochem.* 11:741.

Boyle, P. J. R., and Whitlock, D. G., 1974, The application of a computer controlled microscope to autoradiographs of nerve tissue, *Proceedings of the DECUS Spring Symposium*, pp. 95–99, Digital Equipment User Society, Maynard, Mass.

Boyle, P. J. R., and Whitlock, D. G., 1975. The minicomputer as a microscope accessory, in: *Proceedings of 12th Annual Rocky Mountain Bioengineering and 12th International ISA Biomedical Science Symposium*, pp. 79–84, Instrument Society of America, Pittsburgh.

Cole, M., and Bond, C. P., 1972, Recent advances in automatic image analysis using a television system, *J. Microsc.* 96:89–96 (Part 1).

Cowan, W. M., and Wann, D. F., 1973, A computer system for the measurement of cell and nuclear sizes, *J. Microsc.* 99:331–348 (Part 3).

Dendy, P. P., 1960, A method for the automatic estimation of grain densities in microautoradiography, *Phys. Med. Biol.* 5:131–137.

Duda, R. O., and Hart, P. E., 1973, *Pattern Classification and Scene Analysis*, Wiley, New York.

Dudley, R. A., and Pelc, S. R., 1953, Automatic grain counter assessing quantitatively high resolution autoradiographs, *Nature (London)* 172:992–993.

Garvey, C., Young, J., Simon, W., and Coleman, P. D., 1972, Semiautomatic dendrite tracking and focussing by computer, *Anat. Rec.* 172:314.

Garvey, C. F., Young, J. H., Coleman, P. D., and Simon, W., 1973, Automated three-dimensional dendrite tracking system, *Electroencephalogr. Clin. Neurophysiol.* 35:199–204.

Glaser, E. M., and Van der Loos, H., 1965, A semiautomatic computer microscope for the analysis of neuronal morphology, *IEEE Trans. Biol. Med. Eng.* 12:22–31.

Gullberg, J. E., 1959, Grain counting instrumentation, *Lab. Invest.* 8(1):94–98.

Hueckel, M. H., 1971, An operator which locates edges in digitized pictures, *Assoc. Comput. Mach.* **18**(1):113–125.

Hueckel, M. H., 1973, A local visual operator which recognizes edges and lines, *J. Assoc. Comput. Mach.* **20**(4):634–647.

Howling, D. H., and Fitzgerald, P. J. 1959, The nature, significance and evaluation of the Swartzchild–Villiger effect in photometric procedures, *J. Biophys. Biochem. Cytol.* **6**:313.

Izzo, N. F., and Coles, W., 1962, Blood-cell scanner identifies rare cells, *Electronics*, April 27.

Kopriwa, B. M., and Le Blond, C. P., 1962, Improvements in the coating technique of radioautography, *J. Histochem. Cytochem.* **10**:269–284.

Lajtha, L. G., Oliver, R., Kumatori, T., and Ellis, F., 1958, On the mechanism of radiation affect on DNA synthesis, *Radiat. Res.* **8**:1–16.

Ledley, R. S., 1964, High speed automatic analysis of biomedical pictures, *Science* **146**:216–223.

Mazia, D., Plaut, W. S., and Ellis, G. W., 1955, A method for the quantitative assessment of autoradiographs, *Exp. Cell Res.* **9**:305–312.

Mertz, M., 1969, Silver grain size measurement in autoradiographs using incident and transmitted light, *Histochemie* **17**:128–137.

Potts, A. M., Hodges, D., Shelman, C. B., Fritz, K. J., Levy, N. S., and Mangnall, Y., 1972, Morphology of the primate optic nerve. I. Method and total fiber count, *Invest. Ophthalmol.* **80**:980–988.

Prensky, W., 1971, Automated image analysis in autoradiography, *Exp. Cell Res.* **69**:388–394.

Preston, K., and Norgren, P. E., 1973, Interactive image processor speeds pattern recognition by computer, *Electronics*, October, pp. 89–98.

Reddy, D. R., Davis, W. J., Ohlander, R. B., and Bihary, D. J., 1973, Computer analysis of neuronal structure, in: *Intracellular Staining in Neurobiology* (S. B. Kater, and C. Nicholson, eds.), Springer-Verlag, New York.

Rodgers, A. W., 1961, A simple photometric device for the quantitation of silver grains in autoradiograms of tissue sections, *Exp. Cell Res.* **24**:228–239.

Rodgers, A. W., 1972, Photometric measurements of grain density in autoradiographs, *J. Microsc.* **96**:141–153 (Part 2).

Rodgers, A. W., 1973, *Techniques of Autoradiography*, Elsevier, New York.

Rosenfeld, A., 1969, *Picture Processing by Computer*, Academic Press, New York.

Rosenfeld, A., and Thurston, M., 1971, Edge and curve detection for visual scene analysis, *IEEE Trans.* **C20**:562–569.

Shinn, C. M., and Kline, R. M., 1968, *A Computer Directed System for Measuring Distance between Edges in Optical Images*, Technical Report No. 10, Computer Systems Laboratory, Washington University, St. Louis.

Stein, P. G., Lipkin, L. E., and Shapiro, H. M., 1969, Spectre II: General purpose microscope input for a computer, *Science* **166**:328–333.

Stengel-Rutkowski, S., Gundlach, H. and Zang, K. D., 1974, Quantitative electronic analysis of chromosome autoradiographs using a television image analysing computer, *Exp. Cell Res.* **87**:313–325.

Tolles, W. E., 1959, Methods of automatic quantitation of microautoradiographs, *Lab. Invest.* **8**(1):99–112.

Wann, D. F., and Cowan, W. M., 1972, An image processing system for the analysis of neuroanatomical data, in: *Proceedings of the Computer Image Processing Symposium*, pp. 411–419, University of Missouri, Columbia, Mo.

Wann, D. F., and Grodsky, H. R., 1972, An automatic focussing algorithm for use in the tracking of three dimensional microscope specimens, *Proc. ISA Biomed. Symp.*, pp. 82–90.

Wann, D. F., Woolsey, T. A., LeDierker, M., and Cowan, W. M., 1973, An on-line digital-computer system for the semiautomatic analysis of golgi-impregnated neurons, *IEEE Trans. Biomed. Eng.* 20(4):233–247.

Wann, D. F., Price J. L., Cowan, W. H., and Agulnek, M. A., 1974, An automated system for counting silver grains in autoradiographs, *Brain Res.* 81: 31–58.

8

Tree Analysis of Neuronal Processes

Robert D. Lindsay

1. Introduction

Looking through the microscope at the delicately Golgi-impregnated neuron, one is struck with its remarkable similarity of appearance to the arborization of a tree. The description of size, shape, and density of the dendritic arborization seems to be characteristic for groups of neurons. Neurons have been classified by type using these subjective characteristics derived from observational techniques. However, closer examination of the dendritic branching patterns, reveals continuous structural variation within each neuron type. A knowledge of the design principles for the neuronal processes is fundamental to understanding the functional interaction of neurons.

The structure of a mammalian neuron is very complex. Fibrous processes protrude from the soma and extensively bifurcate. This complex neuronal structure can be mathematically represented by a data model. The *stick* or *wire model* has been most commonly used to represent the bifurcating structure of neuronal processes (see Lindsay, Chapter 1). Several automated data-acquisition techniques have been developed to acquire the structural data using this model and have been described in earlier chapters.

Treating the morphology of neuronal processes as bifurcating treelike structures suggests the measurement of branch lengths and branch angles. Bok (1936, 1959) and Sholl (1956), using visual measurements through the microscope, have studied the branching pattern of dendrites and measured their branch lengths. More recently, Smit *et al.* (1972), Uylings and Smit (1975), and Hollingworth and Berry (1975) have used classical methods to study the branching pattern of neuronal processes and to measure a number of structural parameters. Using modern data-acquisition techniques, Lindsay (1971), Lindsay

---

Robert D. Lindsay · Brain Research Institute and Department of Anatomy, University of California School of Medicine, Los Angeles, California 90024.

and Scheibel (1974, 1976), Chiang (1973), and Paldino (1975) have statistically studied branch lengths and branch angles of neuronal processes in the mammalian central nervous system.

2 *Statistical Methods*

The representation of neuronal processes using the stick data model requires several thousand numbers. Structural measures are easily extracted from the stick data using computer programs. Frequently this data reduction can be accomplished in a general manner, such as computing all branch lengths and branch angles for the structure.

A general approach used to statistically analyze bifurcating neuronal processes has been to select a measure from a group of structural components to form a data set. The data set is considered as a distribution of some measure of the structure, and the mean, variance, standard deviation, and standard deviation of the mean are calculated. The frequency distribution is also determined. An arbitrary theoretical function can be fitted to the experimental distribution, and the "goodness of fit," the chi-square statistic, is calculated.

Two theoretical functions have been used. The first is the *gamma density function* (Clark and Disney, 1970). A continuous random variable x with range $0 < x < \infty$ is said to have a gamma density if its probability density function has the form

$$f(x) = cx^{\beta - 1} e^{-\alpha x} \qquad 0 < x < \infty$$

where α and β are positive constants and c is defined using the gamma function as

$$c = \alpha^{\beta}/\Gamma(\beta)$$

Using the moment-generating function of a random variable having a gamma density, the mean and variance are easily calculated. The mean (μ) and variance (σ^2) are given by the following relationships:

$$\mu = \beta/\alpha \qquad \text{and} \qquad \sigma^2 = \beta/\alpha^2$$

However, the relationships of α and β in terms of μ and σ^2 are more useful for our purposes and are given by

$$\alpha = \mu/\sigma^2 \qquad \text{and} \qquad \beta = \mu^2/\sigma^2$$

For the special case when the constant β is equal to 1, the function becomes the negative exponential density function. A useful theorem in interpreting the negative exponential density function is the following:

> *Theorem I:* Let X be a continuous variable with the range $0 < x < \infty$. For each fixed $s > 0$, assume that, conditional on X being greater than s, the probability density function of $X - s$ is the same as the unconditional probability density function of X. Then X has a negative exponential probability density function. Conversely, any random variable having a negative exponential probability density function has this property (Clark and Disney, 1970).

Another useful theorem in interpreting the gamma density function where β is any integer is the following:

> *Theorem II:* If $X_1, X_2, \ldots, X_\beta$ are independent random variables, each having a negative exponential density with mean $1/\alpha$, then $X = X_1 + \ldots + X_\beta$ will have a gamma density of the form given above (Clark and Disney, 1970).

These theorems have been useful in understanding the results of our analyses.

For ratios of μ^2 to σ^2 larger than 18, the gaussian density function is more convenient as a theoretical function. The gaussian density function has the form

$$f(x) = (1/2\pi\sigma^2)^{1/2} e^{-(x-\mu)^2/2\sigma^2} \qquad -\infty < x < \infty$$

where all parameters are as already defined above.

Once the statistical calculations have been completed and a theoretical function has been determined, the results are printed out by the computer. The computer also plots as a graph the experimental distribution in the form of a histogram and the theoretical density function normalized to the experimental data.

After the set of each measure has been examined, the measures can be paired and examined for functional dependence. A graphic presentation of the paired data in the form of a scattergram is generally useful in guiding the analytical approach. *Correlation analysis* and *regression analysis* are two statistical methods used to attack this kind of problem. Computational methods and FORTRAN subprograms have been developed by Bevington (1969) which are useful in carrying out correlation and regression analysis on the computer.

Another approach has been to consider only the topology of the branching pattern and to ignore all the geometrical components. This formal mathematical treatment of treelike structures is found in the theory of graphs (Harary, 1969). Each neuron process can be classified according to its branching pattern. In addition, each segment or branch in the pattern can be assigned an order. There are several systems used to assign branch orders to a treelike structure. These systems have been reviewed by Berry *et al.* (1975) and Uylings *et al.* (1975).

3. Applications

A number of statistical analysis computer programs have been developed to study the branching pattern of neuronal processes. The branch lengths and branch angles are easily calculated from the stick data. Each dendrite and axon is processed individually. The sequence of the points is scanned for branch and end codes. Fiber lengths between adjacent branch points (called nodes) and lengths between adjacent branch and end points (called termini) are calculated and stored in a two-dimensional array in such a manner as to preserve the topological structure of the process. For each branch point, there are an incoming branch and two outgoing branches. An angle is formed by each outgoing branch and the extended direction of the incoming branch. Thus a branch angle is associated with each outgoing branch of the structure. The angles are also stored in a two-dimensional array. The branch-length and branch-angle arrays are stored on magnetic tape for statistical analysis.

Computer programs for the following structural measures have been developed: soma to first node fiber length; node to node fiber length; node to terminus fiber length; total fiber length; soma to terminus fiber length; soma to last node fiber length; branch angles. For each set of measures, the following statistics were calculated: the number of measures (n); the mean value (μ); the standard deviation of the mean (σ_μ); the standard deviation (σ); the alpha constant of the gamma density function (α); the beta constant of the gamma density function (β); the reduced chi-square statistic from the distribution and the theoretical function (χ^2); the number of degrees of freedom used in the chi-square calculation (ν); the probability of observing a value larger than χ^2 for a random sample of n observations with ν degrees of freedom (ρ). In addition to the statistical calculations, the experimental frequency distribution histograms and theoretical density functions were plotted for each set of structural measures.

The internodal branch lengths, called links, can be divided into groups by assigning a branch order to the links. Since the branching patterns in general are not symmetrical, the ordering of the links can be defined in several ways. Two different schemes were selected to assign branch orders to the links in the asymmetrical bifurcating dendritic structures. The first starts with the initial projection from the soma and continues sequentially numbering the links outward toward the termini. This scheme will be referred to as *centrifugal ordering* (see Fig. 1a). The second scheme orders the links from the termini inward toward the soma. Since the pattern is asymmetrical, inner links may be assigned different orders derived from different termini. The selection is made unique by assigning the largest number as the order of the link (see Fig. 1b). The second scheme is referred to as *centripetal ordering.*

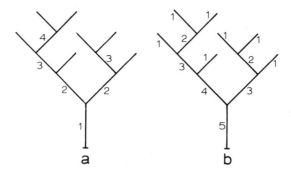

Fig. 1. Diagram of link ordering. (a) Centrifugal. (b) Centripetal.

Another method of presenting the internodal branch length data is in the form of a graph. The mean value of the internodal lengths for each branch order is plotted along the ordinate of the graph. The small cross is the value of the mean, the inner bracket is the standard error of the mean, and the outer bracket is the standard deviation of the distribution. The abscissa value is the branch-order mean value plus the sum of all preceding branch-order mean values. This graph gives a sense of the change of the branching probability as one moves from the soma to the termini for centrifugal ordering and from the termini toward the soma for centripetal ordering.

Branch-order analysis has been applied to basal dendrites of second-layer pyramidal cells. These neurons were selected from the sensory cortex of the adult albino rat. Figures 2 and 3 present the frequency distributions for the internodal lengths for each branch order using the centrifugal and centripetal ordering schemes. Graphs of the branch-order means and standard deviations are plotted for the centrifugal ordering in Fig. 4 and for the centripetal ordering in Fig. 5.

The distributions for two additional measures are presented for the same group of dendritic structures, the soma to terminus length data in Fig. 6 and the branch-angle data in Fig. 7.

Thus far, only measures that are invariant to the choice of the coordinate system used in the representation of the structure have been discussed. There are measures which are dependent on the particular coordinate system chosen. In examining the neuronal structure, the spatial distribution of certain points may be of special interest. The measures in this case would be a coordinate value of the point.

Two types of points, the nodes and termini, have been chosen to illustrate the analysis of these types of measures. The structural data were collected from granular cells of human dentate gyrus. The somata of these cells lie in a thin lamina, and the dendrites of each cell are confined to an inverted cone. A

Robert D. Lindsay

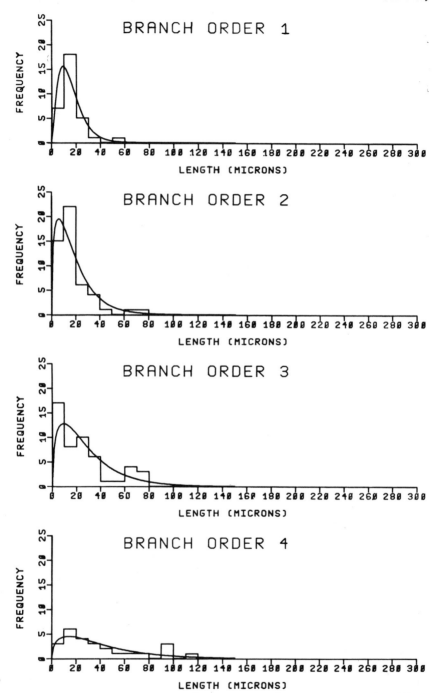

Fig. 2. Distribution of basal dendritic branch lengths using centrifugal ordering.

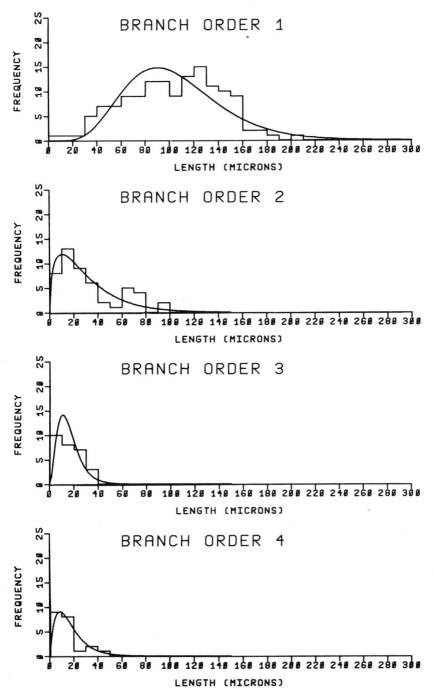

Fig. 3. Distribution of basal dendritic branch lengths using centripetal ordering.

Robert D. Lindsay

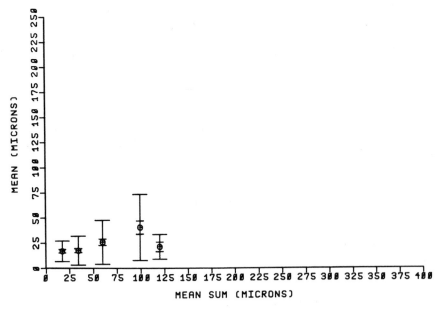

Fig. 4. Graph of basal dendritic branch length means using centripetal ordering.

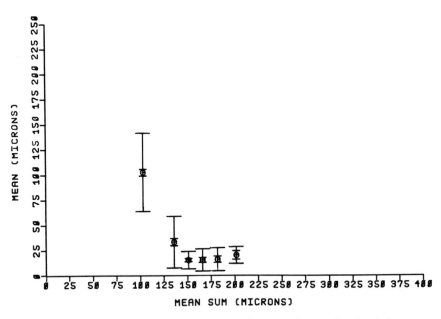

Fig. 5. Graph of basal dendritic branch length means using centripetal ordering.

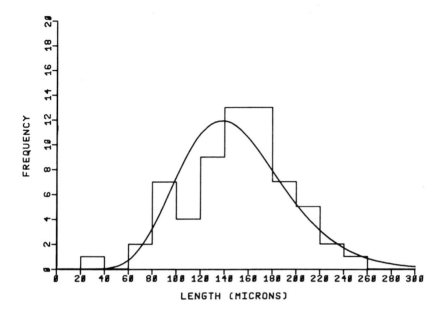

Fig. 6. Distribution of basal dendritic soma to terminus lengths.

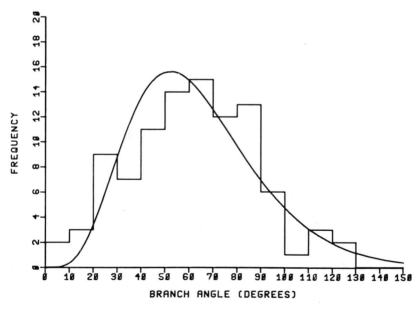

Fig. 7. Distribution of basal dendritic branch angles.

Robert D. Lindsay

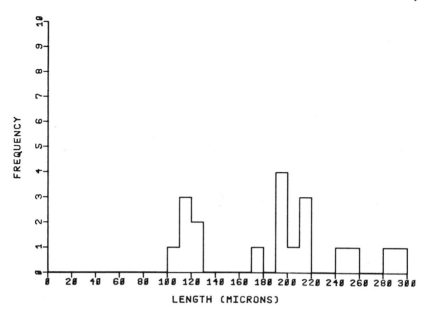

Fig. 8. Histogram of radii for cylinders which enclose the dendritic structure.

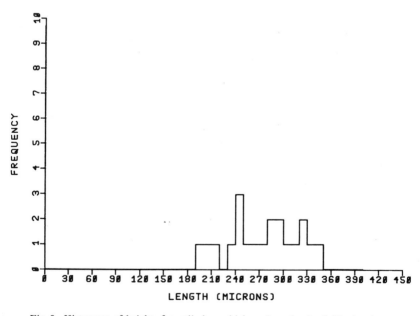

Fig. 9. Histogram of heights for cylinders which enclose the dendritic structure.

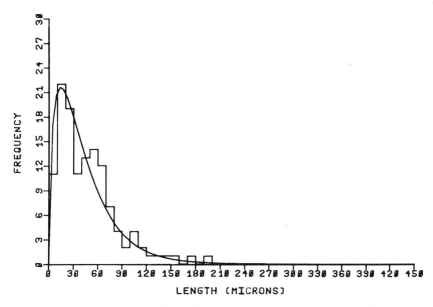

Fig. 10. Distribution of the radii coordinates of branch nodes for granular cell dendrites.

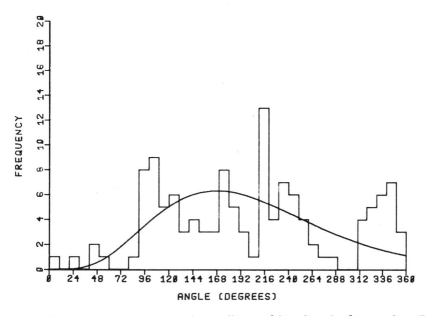

Fig. 11. Distribution of the polar angle coordinates of branch nodes for granular cell dendrites.

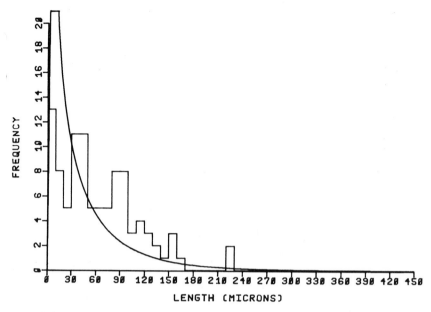

Fig. 12. Distribution of the height coordinates of branch nodes for granular cell dendrites.

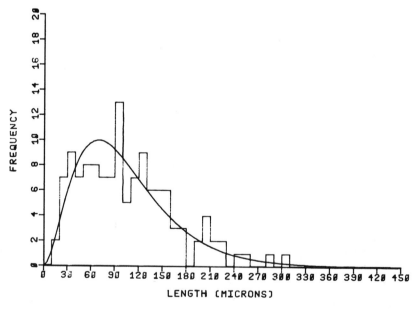

Fig. 13. Distribution of the origin–node lengths for granular cell dendrites.

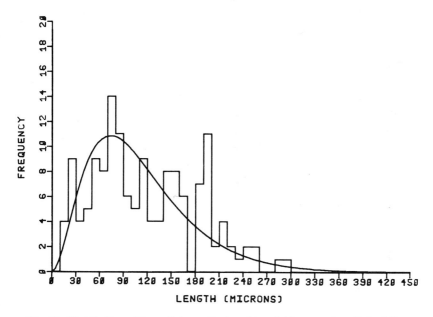

Fig. 14. Distribution of the radial coordinates of termini for granular cell dendrites.

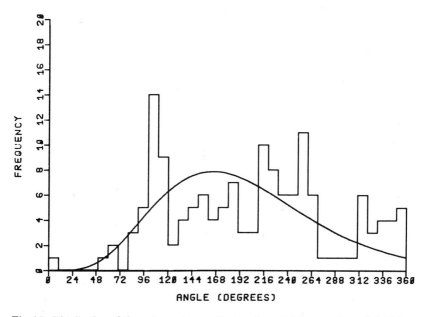

Fig. 15. Distribution of the polar angle coordinates of termini for granular cell dendrites.

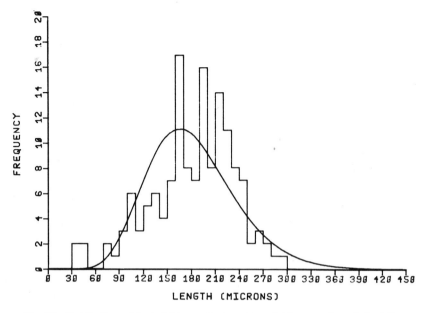

Fig. 16. Distribution of the height coordinates of termini for granular cell dendrites.

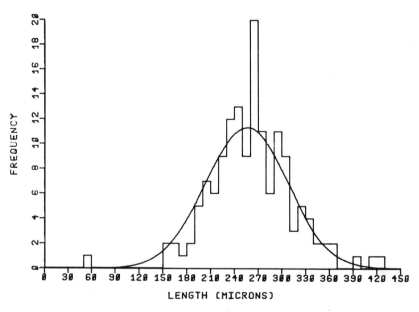

Fig. 17. Distribution of the origin–termini lengths for granular cell dendrites.

cylindrical coordinate system is defined by choosing the origin as the center of the soma and the Z-axis perpendicular to the lamina.

Figures 8 and 9 are histograms of the minimum radius and minimum height, respectively, of a cylinder that encloses the dendritic structure for each neuron in the sample. The cylindrical coordinates, the radius (R), the polar angle (A), the height (Z), and the distance between the origin and the points (S) have been selected as structural measures. The frequency distributions of these measures for the branch nodes and termini are presented in Figs. 10–17. The experimental distributions are fitted with gamma density or gaussian functions. Some of the chi-square values indicate that these functions are inappropriate for these distributions. The challenge is to find appropriate functions and to interpret the geometrical meaning of these functions.

4. Conclusion

There is a remarkable similarity between the structure of bifurcating neuronal processes and the branches of trees. The stick data model has been used to represent quantitatively the structure of bifurcating neuronal processes. Automated data systems have been developed to collect structural data of neuronal processes using the data model. Large amounts of quantitative data collected by these systems suggest the use of statistical analysis.

The general approach has been to extract measures from structural data and to examine the distributions of these measures. Statistical parameters are calculated for each set of measures. The distribution is fitted with a theoretical function. The question of whether the measure under consideration represents stochastic or rigid design is of fundamental importance in the choice of a function. A number of probability density functions may be fitted to the distributions which have a clear interpretation.

The objective of applying statistical methods to neuronal structural data is to develop design principles which relate to the function and development of nervous systems.

ACKNOWLEDGMENTS

The support and the encouragement of the Scheibels have been greatly appreciated. Research by the author was supported by USPHS Grant NS 10657, N.I.N.D.S. The assistance and encouragement of my wife, Barbara, in the preparation of this chapter are gratefully acknowledged.

5. References

Berry, M., Hollingworth, T., Anderson, E. M., and Flinn, R. M., 1975, Application of network analysis to the study of the branching pattern of dendritic fields, in: *Advances in Neurology*, Vol. 12 (G. W. Kreutzberg, ed.), Raven Press, New York.

Bevington, P. R., 1969, *Data Reduction and Error Analysis for the Physical Sciences*, McGraw-Hill, New York.

Bok, S. T., 1936, The branching of dendrites in the cerebral cortex, *Proc. Acad. Sci. (Amsterdam)* **39**:1209–1218.

Bok, S. T., 1959, *Histonomy of the Cerebral Cortex*, Elsevier, Amsterdam.

Chiang, B. S., 1973, The organization of the visual cortex, dissertation, Physics Department, Syracuse University.

Clark, A. B., and Disney, R. L., 1970, *Probability and Random Processes for Engineers and Scientists*, Wiley, New York.

Harary, F., 1969, *Graph Theory*, Addison-Wesley, Reading, Mass.

Hollingworth, T., and Berry, M., 1975, Network analysis of dendritic fields of pyramidal cells in neocortex and Purkinje cells in the cerebellum of the rat, *Philos. Trans. R. Soc. London Ser. B* **270**:227–262.

Lindsay, R. D., 1971, Connectivity of the cerebral cortex, dissertation, Physics Department, Syracuse University.

Lindsay, R. D., and Scheibel, A. B., 1974, Quantitative analysis of the dendritic branching pattern of small pyramidal cells from adult rat somesthetic and visual cortex, *Exp. Neurol.* **45**:424–434.

Lindsay, R. D., and Scheibel, A. B., 1976, Quantitative analysis of dendritic branch pattern of granular cells from human dentate gyrus, *Exp. Neurol.* **52**:295–310.

Paldino, A. M., 1975, A computerized study of the axonal structure in the visual cortex, dissertation, Physics Department, Syracuse University.

Sholl, D. A., 1956, *The Organization of the Cerebral Cortex*, Methuen, London.

Smit, G. J., Uylings, H. B. M., and Veldmaat-Wansink, L., 1972, The branching pattern in dendrites of cortical neurons, *Acta Morphol. Neerl. Scand.* **9**:253–274.

Uylings, H. B. M., and Smit, G. J., 1975, Three-dimensional branching structure of pyramid cell dendrites, *Brain Res.* **87**:55–60.

Uylings, H. B. M., Smit, G. J., and Veltman, W. A. M., 1975, Ordering methods in quantitative analysis of branching structures of dendritic trees, in: *Advances in Neurology*, Vol. 12 (G. W. Kreutzberg, ed.), Raven Press, New York.

9

Neuronal Field Analysis Using Fourier Series

Robert D. Lindsay

1. Introduction

Most mammalian neurons have very complex structures. Fibrous processes protrude from the somata and extensively bifurcate to form arborizations similar in nature to the structure of a tree. Data models have been developed which approximate these complex structures to within a certain degree of resolution. The data model most commonly used to represent the bifurcating structure of neuronal processes is the *stick* or *wire model* (Lindsay, Chapter 1). Automated data-acquisition techniques have been developed to acquire the structural data for this model. Several detailed descriptions of systems for data acquisition have been presented in earlier chapters of this volume.

Two general quantitative analysis schemes have been applied to the structural data collected with these systems. The first scheme is to treat the morphology of the neuronal processes as bifurcating treelike structures. The focus of this method is on the individual branches and their position in the topology of the fibrous structure. This scheme has been discussed in detail in an earlier chapter (Lindsay, Chapter 8).

The second general analysis scheme is to treat the neuronal structure as a fiber density field. In this approach, variables associated with the overall geometry of the neuronal processes are of interest. Variables associated with individual branches will not be of concern. One variable of interest is the fiber surface area per unit volume in space. The objective of the method is to obtain an analytical function that expresses the average density of fiber surface area at a point in space. The transformation of a discrete segmented function to an analytical function is a familiar problem in applied mathematics. The most common method for this type of transformation utilizes the Fourier series.

Robert D. Lindsay · Brain Research Institute and Department of Anatomy, University of California School of Medicine, Los Angeles, California 90024.

2. Derivation

An arbitrary function $f(x)$, given for $a \leqslant x \leqslant b$, has a representation as a Fourier series over the interval. In some problems, it may be advantageous to represent the function by the corresponding series. That is, given a function $f(x)$, it may be expanded as

$$f(x) = A_0/2 + \sum_{n=1}^{\infty} (A_n \cos ns + B_n \sin nx) \qquad (1)$$

where

$$A_n = \frac{1}{\pi} \int_{-\pi}^{\pi} f(x) \cos nx \, dx \qquad (n = 0,1,2, \ldots) \qquad (2)$$

and

$$B_n = \frac{1}{\pi} \int_{-\pi}^{\pi} f(x) \sin nx \, dx \qquad (n = 1,2,3, \ldots) \qquad (3)$$

and where the independent variable has been transformed so that $(-\pi,\pi)$ is the desired interval.

The first term in the series is a constant and is equal to the mean value of the function $f(x)$ in the interval $(-\pi,\pi)$. The means of all the other terms in the interval are equal to zero. These additional terms added to the constant term do not change the mean value of the series, but add more resolution in approximating the function $f(x)$ by adding to certain pieces of the interval and equally subtracting from other pieces of the interval. Mathematically, one says that the series uniformly converges to the function as more and more terms are included in the summation.

The theory of Fourier series can be generalized with minor changes to functions of several variables (Kaplan, 1952). The interval is replaced by a bounded closed region R and the definite integral by a multiple integral over R. An arbitrary function $f(x,y,z)$, given for $-\pi \leqslant x \leqslant \pi$, $-\pi \leqslant y \leqslant \pi$, and $-\pi \leqslant z \leqslant \pi$, has a representation as a Fourier series over the region. The function may be expanded as

$$
\begin{aligned}
f(x, y, z) = \sum_{l=0}^{\infty} \sum_{m=0}^{\infty} \sum_{n=0}^{\infty} \Big(& SSS_{lmn} \cdot \sin lx \cdot \sin my \cdot \sin nz \\
& + CSS_{lmn} \cdot \cos lx \cdot \sin my \cdot \sin nz \\
& + SCS_{lmn} \cdot \sin lx \cdot \cos my \cdot \sin nz \\
& + CCS_{lmn} \cdot \cos lx \cdot \cos my \cdot \sin nz \\
& + SSC_{lmn} \cdot \sin lx \cdot \sin my \cdot \cos nz \\
& + CSC_{lmn} \cdot \cos lx \cdot \sin my \cdot \cos nz \\
& + SCC_{lmn} \cdot \sin lx \cdot \cos my \cdot \cos nz \\
& + CCC_{lmn} \cdot \cos lx \cdot \cos my \cdot \cos nz \Big)
\end{aligned} \qquad (4)
$$

where

$$SSS_{lmn} = \iiint_R f(x, y, z) \sin lx \cdot \sin my \cdot \sin nz \, dx \, dy \, dz \qquad (5)$$

and similarly for the other coefficients of the series.

The structure of the neuronal processes may be represented as a series of connected straight lines. By transforming this discrete structure using a Fourier series, one can obtain a density function which is continuous and smooth in a defined region of space. The density function of most interest is the membrane surface area per unit volume in space. To simplify the analysis, the fiber length per unit volume in space will be developed in detail. The relationship between membrane area and fiber length densities is a multiplicative constant if one approximates the fiber diameter by an average value. The expansion of the method to include varying diameters does not introduce any fundamental changes in the analysis, but does introduce a greater degree of complexity.

The direct application of equations like (5) to obtain the expansion coefficients for a sticklike structure is very difficult. The structure consists of a series of connected tubes in space. The function is equal to unity within the volume of the tube and zero everywhere else. Usually one would set up this kind of a problem using the limits of integration to include only the finite part of the function. Using this procedure for the tubular structures leads to very complex expressions. A simpler procedure takes advantage of its tubular or linelike structure. Instead of integrating over all space in the region, one integrates along the line that represents the structure. Thus the multiple integral over three-dimensional space in the region can be reduced to a single integral along the line representing the structure.

The reduction of the multiple integral is accomplished by choosing a parameter and finding the functional relationship between the parameter and the independent variables, substituting these functions for the independent variables and integrating the resultant function between appropriate limits. Since the function is a series of connected straight-line segments, the natural selection for the parameter is the unit length along the segment. Each line segment is transformed to a definite integral. The sum of these integrals is equal to the original multiple integral integrated over the entire structure.

The functional relationships between the x, y, z coordinates and the unit length (t) along the line segment are given by

$$x = x_1 + \alpha \cdot t \qquad (6)$$

$$y = y_1 + \beta \cdot t \qquad (7)$$

$$z = z_1 + \gamma \cdot t \qquad (8)$$

where (x_1, y_1, z_1) is the initial end point of the line segment and α, β, γ are respectively the direction cosines. The limits of integration are from zero to the length of the line segment.

The development of the Fourier series analysis technique has been described for a rectangular system. Sometimes, the structure of a problem suggests that simpler relationships may exist if a different coordinate system is used. Such is the case for the dendritic arborization of neurons. Many neurons have a cylindrical or spherical symmetry. To extend the analysis to cylindrical or spherical coordinate systems, the independent variables x, y, z in equations (4) and (5) are replaced by r, ϕ, z for the cylindrical case and r, ϕ, θ for the spherical case. The multiple integrals are reduced using the same parametric method with the addition of the functional relationships between the x, y, z variables and the r, ϕ, z or r, ϕ, θ variables. These functions are given by

$$r = (x^2 + y^2)^{1/2} \tag{9}$$

$$\phi = \arctan(y/x) \tag{10}$$

$$z = z \tag{11}$$

for the cylindrical case, and

$$r = (x^2 + y^2 + z^2)^{1/2} \tag{12}$$

$$\phi = \arctan(y/x) \tag{13}$$

$$\theta = \arctan[z/(x^2 + y^2 + z^2)^{1/2}] \tag{14}$$

for the spherical case. The coefficients in the series using cylindrical or spherical coordinates reflect structural parameters relative to an axis through the structure.

3. Application

The Fourier series analysis technique was developed in a form to be applied directly to the stick data model of neuronal processes. The application of the technique using the cylindrical coordinate system will now be discussed in detail. The technique generates two products — the coefficients, which have geometrical meaning, and the series, which is an analytical function representing the structure.

In setting up the problem for a neuron, one chooses an origin and an axis through the structure. Also, a cylinder is chosen which encases the structure. The center of the soma is selected as the origin of the coordinate system. Values for the radius and height are determined that represent the smallest cylinder which encases the structure. The radius and the height of this cylinder are used to normalize the r coordinate to the range from 0 to 2π and the z coordinate to the range from $-\pi$ to π.

When any of the indices in equation (4) is equal to zero, there is a reduction in the complexity of the associated term in the series. If the index equal to zero is associated with the SIN function, then the corresponding coefficient is equal to zero, and the term need not be considered in the series. Also, if the index equal to zero is associated with the COS function, then the corresponding COS function is equal to one and the complexity of the term is reduced.

When all the indices are equal to zero, the only nonzero term in the series is $CCC_{000} \cdot 1 \cdot 1 \cdot 1$, which is equal to the total fiber length of the structure in the cylindrical volume. When two of the three indices are equal to zero, a set of terms results with a dependence on a single variable. The associated coefficients represent the structural dependence on this variable with an average contribution from the other variables. When one of the three indices is equal to zero, a set of terms results with a dependency on two variables. These associated coefficients represent the structural correlation of the two variables.

The Fourier series analysis technique using a cylindrical coordinate system was applied to three sticklike structures to illustrate the method. Diagrams of the structures are shown in Fig. 1. The circles have a radius of 2π and all lines lie in the $z = 0$ plane.

The following trigonometric relationship is useful in interpreting the geometric meaning of the coefficients:

$$a \sin (\theta) + b \cos (\theta) = A \cos (\theta + \theta^0)$$

where $A = (a^2 + b^2)^{1/2}$ and $\theta^0 = \arctan (a/b)$. The SIN and COS terms for a single variable and the same harmonic (same value of n) may be combined into a single term where the two coefficients have been transformed to an amplitude

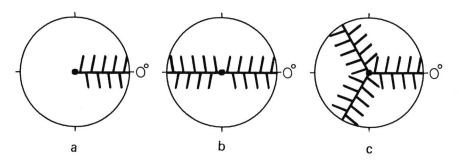

a   b   c

Fig. 1. Diagram of three stick structures. All the structures are in the X-Y plane at $z = 0$. The radius of each circle is 2π. (a) Monopolar structure. (b) Bipolar structure. (c) Tripolar structure.

(*A*) and a phase angle (θ°) (see Jenkins and White, 1957, for a derivation of this result).

In Fig. 2, the amplitudes for the terms containing a single variable have been presented for the three structures of Fig. 1. The amplitudes associated with functions of *r* are related to the localization of the fiber density in concentric cylinders about the *Z*-axis. The amplitudes for harmonic functions of *r* do not indicate any localization of the fiber density in the *r* dimension.

The amplitudes associated with the functions of φ are related to the localization of the fiber density in planes parallel to the *Z* axis and intersecting the *Z* axis. The functions of φ form a set of polar configurations. The order of the harmonic determines the number of the poles evenly spaced around the *Z* axis, and hence the amplitude for each harmonic function of φ is related to the overlap of the structure and the polar configuration. The relationship between the polar configuration and the amplitudes is not a direct one, but is dependent on the sequence of the amplitudes. The repetition of the major contributing amplitudes is directly related to the polar configuration as is demonstrated in Fig. 2.

The amplitudes associated with the functions of *z* are related to the localization of the fiber density to planes which are perpendicular to the *Z* axis. The three structures in Fig. 1 represent a simple case; that is, all of the fibers lie in a single plane through the origin. The amplitudes for the harmonic functions of *z* are all of significant value, indicating that the structure is highly structured in the *z* dimension. The fact that the amplitudes are equal in value further indicates that the structure is confined to a single plane. When the structure is more dispersed in the *z* dimension, then the amplitudes decrease in value as the order increases.

The coefficients associated with the SIN and COS functions for each harmonic were combined to form an amplitude and a phase angle. The phase angles are also useful in interpreting the geometric meaning of the coefficients. Consider the phase angles for the functions of φ. The value of the phase angle is the angle to which the first pole is directed. For each of the structures in Fig. 1, the first pole is directed along the φ = 0 line. If the structures were rotated about the *Z* axis by an angle φ°, then the phase angles would be equal to φ°. The phase angles combine with the amplitudes to indicate the amount of localization, but they also directly indicate the position of the localization along the coordinate axis.

When the series is summed with a large number of terms, the function begins to approximate the treelike structure. Since the structure of neuronal processes appears stochastic for many types of neurons (Lindsay, 1971; Lindsay and Scheibel, 1974, 1976; Chiang, 1973; Paldino, 1975), a function which averages the amount of branch length over space might be useful in assessing the gross structure of axonal and dendritic fields. Indeed, the geometric parameters

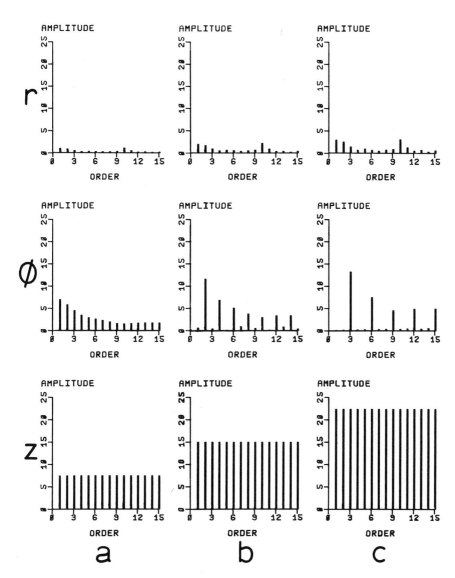

Fig. 2. Bar graphs of the single-variable coefficients. (a) Monopolar structure. (b) Bipolar structure. (c) Tripolar structure.

generated are related to the descriptive language used in classical morphology. It has already been stated that the series has the same mean value over the region regardless of where the series is terminated. Hence for a series of low order the function represents a treelike structure averaged out over space, but still preserving its average value.

The graphic presentation of this density function may be accomplished in several ways. First, the functional relationship to a single variable may be plotted as a graph where all but the one variable have been set equal to constants. Figure 3 is an example of one of these single-variable presentations. The second method

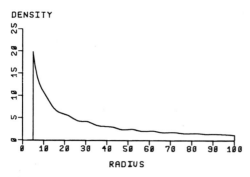

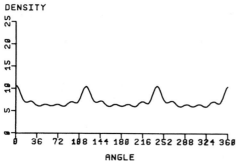

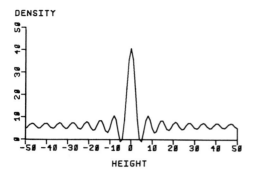

Fig. 3. Graphs of fiber density as a function of the radius, the polar angle, and the height for the tripolar structure. Only the constant term and the single-variable terms have been included. The function has not been normalized to a density; only functional dependence is intended.

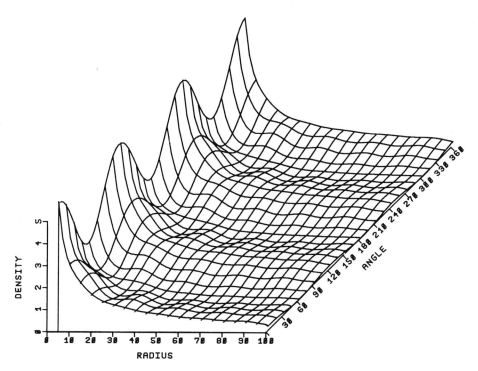

Fig. 4. Surface plot of fiber density as a function of the radius and polar angle for the tripolar structure. The function has not been normalized to a density; only functional dependence is intended.

is to present the density function as a surface by setting one variable equal to a constant. Figure 4 is an example of this method. The third method is to contour the function. Although the computer techniques have been developed (Lindsay, unpublished), our present computer hardware configuration is not capable of carrying out the generation of the graphic presentation in any reasonable amount of time. However, the graphic presentation using this idea is presented in Fig. 5.

A Fourier series is not the only series that can be used to represent an arbitrary function. There are other functions besides the SIN and COS that can be used. These functions are a special example of a general class of functions known as orthogonal sets of functions. Some of the more common examples of these sets of functions used in physics are Bessel functions, Legendre functions, confluent hypergeometric functions, and Hermite functions (Margenau and Murphy, 1956; Arfken, 1966).

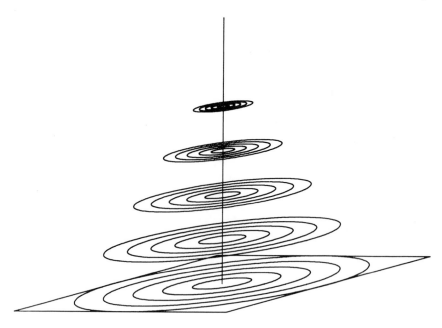

Fig. 5. Contour plot of a three-dimensional density function.

4. Conclusion

Considering the arborization of neuronal processes as a field is not a new idea. Donald Sholl (1956) postulated that overlapping dendritic and axonal fields are proportional to neuronal connectivity. Braitenberg and Lauria (1960) have assigned geometric shapes to the axonal and dendritic patterns for several types of neurons and made estimates of the geometric parameters. However, they considered only the overlap of the shapes. The extension of a shape to a field requires the representation of the neuronal processes as a density function.

The structure of neuronal processes can be represented by the stick data model. Data-acquisition techniques have been developed to collect structural data using this model. The stick data can be transformed to a fiber density function using Fourier series analysis. The coefficients of the series have geometric meaning. The fiber density function generated by the Fourier series can be graphically presented in several forms.

This analysis technique treats the neuronal processes as a field and is primarily intended for use with parameters associated with the overall geometry of the neuronal processes.

ACKNOWLEDGMENTS

The support and the encouragement of the Scheibels have been greatly appreciated. Research by the author was supported by USPHS Grant 10657, N.I.N.D.S. The assistance and encouragement of my wife, Barbara, in the preparation of this chapter are gratefully acknowledged.

5. *References*

Arfken, G., 1966, *Mathematical Methods for Physicists*, Academic Press, New York.

Braitenberg, V., and Lauria, F. E., 1960, Toward a mathematical description of grey substance of nervous system, *Nuovo Cin.* **18**:149–165 (Suppl. 2).

Chiang, B. S., 1973, The organization of the visual cortex, dissertation, Physics Department, Syracuse University.

Jenkins, F. A., and White, H. E., 1957, *Fundamentals of Optics*, McGraw-Hill, New York.

Kaplan, W., 1952, *Advanced Calculus*, Addison-Wesley, Reading, Mass.

Lindsay, R. D., 1971, Connectivity of the cerebral cortex, dissertation, Physics Department, Syracuse University.

Lindsay, R. D., and Scheibel, A. B., 1974, Quantitative analysis of the dendritic branching pattern of small pyramidal cells from adult rat somesthetic and visual cortex, *Exp. Neurol.* **45**:424–434.

Lindsay, R. D., and Scheibel, A. B., 1976, Quantitative analysis of dendritic branching pattern of granular cells from human dentate gyrus, *Exp. Neurol.* **52**:295–310.

Margenau, H., and Murphy, G. M., 1956, *The Mathematics of Physics and Chemistry*, Van Nostrand, Princeton, N.J.

Paldino, A. M., 1975, A computerized study of axonal structure in the visual cortex, dissertation, Physics Department, Syracuse University.

Sholl, D., 1956, *The Organization of the Cerebral Cortex*, Methuen, London.

10

Neuron Orientations: A Computer Application

Christopher Brown

1. Introduction

Does rearing kittens in highly structured visual environments result in differences of physical configuration in individual neurons which correlate with other observed changes in neural characteristics [such as the orientation of their visual fields (Hubel and Wiesel, 1962)]? This question is under investigation, with the physical parameter in question being the "orientation" of the dendritic field of the neuron. In this chapter, computer-based techniques are outlined for acquisition and representation of relevant data, and for describing "orientation" quantitatively.

Kittens are reared in environments with visual limitations such as vertical or horizontal black-and-white stripes. Sections of their brains are stained to render neural dendrites visible, and microscope slides of the sections are prepared. At this point, the computer becomes useful in data acquisition. Garvey *et al*. (1973) describe an automated dendrite tracker which consists of a minicomputer controlling the stage and focus of a microscope and also interfaced to a Vidissector which looks down the microscope. Input from the Vidissector is used to track the dendrites. A tracking spot is superimposed on a screen showing the microscope's field of view, and an operator positions this spot at the base of a dendrite. The dendrite-tracking program then automatically follows the stained dendrite through the brain section in three dimensions. To do this, it follows the dendrite at a given focus by moving the microscope stage, keeping the tracking spot centered on the dendrite; when the dendrite leaves the shallow plane of microscope focus, the tracker refocuses the

---

Christopher Brown • Department of Computer Science, University of Rochester, Rochester, New York 14627.

microscope to restore the image quality. Thus by monitoring the compensations in stage position and focus which were needed to follow the dendrite, and by applying appropriate calibration calculations, the tracker builds up an internal model of what it has seen; it can remember the total length of dendrite followed and has a three-dimensional "wire tree" description of where it has been. This tree is a structure of straight ("wire") segments which may change direction or bifurcate. (Figure 1 shows two wire trees in two dimensions.)

The tracker at present is not entirely automatic, but is overseen by an operator. When the tracker encounters a situation in which the correct direction to take is in doubt (e.g., when two branches cross at a small angle and both branches are fairly well in focus), it halts and asks for advice. This interactive mode of operation is representative of many applications in which the computer routinely performs tedious perceptual and/or arduous bookkeeping tasks, but which now and then demand a more complex perceptual act or strategic decision.

Since the orientation of neurons relative to the cortical surface is in question, the coordinate axes which must be used vary over a section of brain. By using the apical dendrite as an indicator of the direction normal to the cortical surface, the data can be put into a "brain-centered" coordinate system that has biological relevance, as opposed to the accidental system imposed by the angle of the sectioning knife. This transformation is done by multiplying the x, y, z points which specify the end points of wire sections by a 3 x 3 matrix specifying a rotation in 3-space.

2. Description of Orientation

The dendrites of a neuron are a three-dimensional structure, occupying a volume; the representations of volumes in a computer in such a form as to render possible the jobs that naturally come to mind (drawing them from various angles, recognizing other instances of them, computing some of their physical properties, deciding how to construct them, etc.) still remain a challenging problem for all shapes but the mathematically simplest. However, if "orientation" is taken to mean simply "direction," then its computer representation is clear. Two questions arise: first, is this definition of orientation rich enough for dendritic fields; second, if it is, how is it to be defined? Herein we *assume* that the answer to the first question is "yes," and we describe a particular answer to the second question.

The definition of orientation we use is that given by "principal-components" analysis of the wire tree data. The idea behind principal components is well known to physicists, who use it to compute "moments of

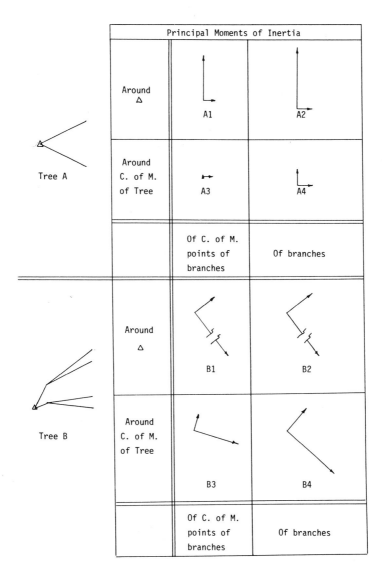

Fig. 1. Principal moments of inertia for two trees. The shortest vector in each points along and gives the error of the best-fit line (and hyperplane, in this two-dimensional case).

inertia," as well as to statisticians, whose name for it we have borrowed. The physicist's and statistician's models differ, however, and part of the goal of this chapter is to repeat a classical result that gives yet a third way to interpret principal components, and relates all three interpretations. This third interpretation is that they provide best-fit lines and planes to three-dimensional data (Pearson, 1901).

Principal-components analysis yields extremely compact descriptions of arbitrarily complicated structures. The descriptors seem apt for at least one sort of orientation, although they do have some questionable features (perhaps most notably the inflexible use of squared distance, in the dispersion/error measure). The description provided typically consists of a point in space which is taken as the "origin" of the structure (often its center of mass), a set of orthogonal axes, or "principal directions," one of which points along (normal to) the best-fit line (plane), and a set of numbers, one associated with each axis direction, that characterize the dispersion about each axis (about the plane normal to that axis). In 3-space, there are thus six numbers which describe the orientation of the structure. Two of the orthogonal axis directions give the third, and, for each of those two directions, two of its direction cosines give the third. We can normalize one dispersion number to unity by dividing all three dispersions by it; the resulting two dispersion ratios make up the total of six numbers. If we wish to keep some measure of the absolute dispersion, all three dispersions are remembered and one more number is needed. To locate the structure in space, three more numbers expressing the origin are needed. Compared with other descriptions of three-dimensional bodies, this representation is quite parsimonious, and, should it prove sufficient for the application, it represents quite an economical choice. After presenting some results which show how to find principal components, in the language of best-fit lines and planes, we shall discuss some modifications and extensions to the method which may be used to enhance the descriptions in a neurophysiological context.

2.1. Derivations and a Classical Result

In what follows, certain notation is used for concise representation of operations on vector components. When it is convenient, vectors are treated as matrices and *vice versa*, and 1×1 matrices are treated as scalars. If $\mathbf{v}$ is a row 3-vector, we use $\partial e / \partial \mathbf{v}$ to indicate the vector $(\partial e / \partial v_1, \partial e / \partial v_2, \partial e / \partial v_3)$. Scalars ($1 \times 1$ matrices) are represented by lowercase italic letters, vectors (row and column matrices) by boldface lowercase letters, $n \times n$ matrices by capital italic letters, the scalar (dot) product of vectors by a $\cdot$, and the transpose of vectors (matrices) by a superscript T.

Consider the problem of finding a plane which "best fits" a swarm of weighted points. If the points are in n-space, the plane is a hyperplane; we will refer to it as a plane. Represent k weighted points in n-space by row n-vectors $\mathbf{x}_i$, $i = 1, 2, \ldots, k$; let the weight of the ith point be w_i. Represent an $(n-1)$-dimensional subspace Π of n-space [a (hyper)plane] by a unit n-vector $\mathbf{z}$ normal to Π and a point $\mathbf{v}$ in Π. In the sequel, all summations run from 1 to k.

The signed perpendicular distance from $\mathbf{x}_i$ to Π is

$$d_{i\Pi} = (\mathbf{x}_i - \mathbf{v}) \cdot \mathbf{z}$$

The error measure we wish to minimize is the sum over all points of the square of this distance times the weight (mass) of the point, i.e.,

$$e = \sum_i [(\mathbf{x}_i - \mathbf{v}) \cdot \mathbf{z}]^2 w_i = \sum_i \mathbf{z}(\mathbf{x}_i - \mathbf{v})^T (\mathbf{x}_i - \mathbf{v}) \mathbf{z}^T w_i = \mathbf{z} M \mathbf{z}^T \qquad (1)$$

In equation (1), M is a real, symmetrical $n \times n$ matrix, sometimes called the "scatter matrix" of the points:

$$M = \sum_i w_i (\mathbf{x}_i - \mathbf{v})^T (\mathbf{x}_i - \mathbf{v}) \qquad (2)$$

First, we show that the best-fit plane passes through the center of mass (C. of M.) of the points.

Proposition 1: For e of equation (1) to be minimized, the plane must pass through the C. of M. of the point swarm. Thus, in equation (1), e attains a minimum when $\mathbf{v}$ is the C. of M.

Proof:

$$e = \sum_i w_i \mathbf{z} (\mathbf{x}_i \cdot \mathbf{x}_i) \mathbf{z}^T - 2 \sum_i w_i \mathbf{z} (\mathbf{x}_i \cdot \mathbf{v}) \mathbf{z}^T + \sum_i w_i \mathbf{z} (\mathbf{v} \cdot \mathbf{v}) \mathbf{z}^T$$

Since $\mathbf{z}\mathbf{z}^T = 1$ by definition,

$$\frac{\partial e}{\partial \mathbf{v}} = -2 \sum_i w_i \mathbf{x}_i + \mathbf{v} \sum_i w_i$$

and setting $\partial e / \partial \mathbf{v} = 0$ implies

$$\mathbf{v} = \frac{\sum_i w_i \mathbf{x}_i}{\sum_i w_i}$$

which is the center of mass.

Thus it is possible to find a point in the best-fit plane. The plane would be determined completely if a normal vector for it could be obtained. This is done next, by the same technique.

Proposition 2: For e of equation (1) to be minimized, $\mathbf{z}$ must be the eigenvector of M with smallest eigenvalue.

Proof: From equation (1),

$$e = \mathbf{z}M\mathbf{z}^T$$

Since $\mathbf{z}\mathbf{z}^T = 1$, $e = \mathbf{z}M\mathbf{z}^T - m(\mathbf{z}\mathbf{z}^T - 1)$ for an undetermined multiplier m. Since M is symmetrical,

$$\frac{\partial e}{\partial \mathbf{z}} = 2\mathbf{z}M - 2\mathbf{z}m$$

and equating this derivative component by component to zero gives

$$\mathbf{z}M = \mathbf{z}m$$

and thus $\mathbf{z}$ is an eigenvector of M. Further, since

$$e = \mathbf{z}M\mathbf{z}^T = \mathbf{z}m\mathbf{z}^T = m$$

then e is minimized when $\mathbf{z}$ is the eigenvector of smallest eigenvalue m.

The plane is now completely determined by $\mathbf{z}$ and $\mathbf{v}$, but it might more conveniently be represented by its plane equation, which of course is derivable from them by applying the following general rule.

Proposition 3: If $\mathbf{v}$ is a point in a plane Π and $\mathbf{z}$ is a unit vector normal to Π, the equation for Π in variables a_i is

$$z_1 a_1 + z_2 a_2 + z_3 a_3 + \cdots + z_n a_n - \mathbf{v} \cdot \mathbf{z} = 0 \tag{3}$$

Proof: For any point $\mathbf{x}$ on Π, $(\mathbf{z} \cdot \mathbf{x})$ is a constant, the distance along $\mathbf{z}$ from Π to the origin. Using this fact with the formal point $\mathbf{a}$ and the point $\mathbf{v}$ known to be in Π yields $\mathbf{z} \cdot \mathbf{a} = \mathbf{z} \cdot \mathbf{v}$, which may be rewritten as equation (3).

Using Propositions 1, 2, and 3, a best-fit plane to a swarm of points may be determined and its plane equation written. Now we turn to perhaps a more familiar concept, that of the moment of inertia of the point swarm around an axis. It so happens that the moment calculations and those for the best-fit plane are closely related.

The matrix M of equation (2) may be written out explicitly; for one point of mass w at $\mathbf{x}$, it is

$$M_x = w \begin{bmatrix} x_1{}^2 & x_1 x_2 & x_1 x_3 & \cdots \\ x_2 x_1 & x_2{}^2 & x_2 x_3 & \cdots \\ x_3 x_1 & x_3 x_2 & x_3{}^2 & \cdots \end{bmatrix}$$

For comparison, here is the "inertia tensor" for the same point. It can be used to compute the moment of inertia of the point around any axis direction.

$$
I_x = w \begin{bmatrix} x_2{}^2 + x_3{}^2 + \cdots + x_n{}^2 & -x_1 x_2 & -x_1 x_3 & \cdots \\ -x_2 x_1 & x_1{}^2 + x_3{}^2 + \cdots + x_n{}^2 & -x_2 x_3 & \cdots \\ -x_3 x_1 & -x_3 x_2 & x_1{}^2 + x_2{}^2 + x_4{}^2 + \cdots + x_n{}^2 & \cdots \\ \cdot & \cdot & & \end{bmatrix}
$$

Both M and I are defined for a swarm of points to be the sum of the M_x or I_x for each point in the swarm. Further, both M and I may be defined for continuous mass distributions by integration instead of summation.

The definition of the moment of inertia of a point around an axis is the square of its distance from the axis times its mass. This is an exact parallel to the definition of error we adopted above, only it is defined relative to a line, the axis. We have shown that, of the eigenvectors of M, the one of smallest eigenvalue is the normal to Π, the hyperplane which minimizes $\Sigma_i w_i d_{i\,\Pi}^2$.

It is therefore perhaps not surprising to us, and it is well known to physicists, that, of the eigenvectors of I, the one of smallest eigenvalue is the direction of the line Λ, the "principal axis" which minimizes $\Sigma_i w_i d_{i\Lambda}^2$, where $d_{i\Lambda}$ is the distance from a point at $\mathbf{x}_i$ to Λ.

Further, the following pretty result is perhaps unfamiliar, because in the usual applications M and I do not both have a meaningful interpretation (although M is sometimes said to measure "inertia about a plane").

Proposition 4: (Karl Pearson) If M and I are computed for the same weighted points, then the eigenvectors of M are the same as those of I, and the vector of minimum eigenvalue of one matrix is the vector of maximum eigenvalue of the other. In fact, if v_M is the eigenvalue for an eigenvector of M and v_I is the eigenvalue for the corresponding eigenvector of I, then

$$
v_M = \frac{\text{trace}(I)}{n-1} - v_I
$$

$$
v_I = \text{trace}(M) - v_M
$$

Thus there is a duality between the best-fit plane and the best-fit line; the best-fit plane lies normal to the major "principal axis" of the inertia ellipsoid defined by **I**.

For example, to compute the best fit line or plane for a point swarm in 3-space, the C. of M. is found first, and then the eigenvalues and eigenvectors of M may be computed by any one of a number of methods (Businger, 1965). If there are $n - 1$ small and one large eigenvalue, the point swarm is "linelike" and the eigenvector of large eigenvalue points along the best-fit line. If there are $n - 1$ large and one small eigenvalue, the swarm is "planelike" and the eigenvector of small value points along the normal to the best-fit plane. Both the best-fit line and plane go through the C. of M. of the points.

Calculation using the inertia matrices instead of scatter matrices is often useful: the idea of moment of inertia of a solid body is well understood, and since I has been computed for several common shapes it is possible to use those results to gain easy answers for continuous mass distributions, converting to best-fit plane terminology via Proposition 4. An example of this technique is given in Section 2.2.

2.2. Extensions and Refinements

In the preceding derivations, point swarms were considered, although the possibility of dealing with continuous distributions was mentioned. One extension to the above method is to characterize the inertia tensor for an actual wire tree, using the known properties of the moments of inertia, i.e., for ideal, straight, one-dimensional continuous mass distributions. A coordinate system is first chosen for the tree. For a wire of length $2d$ and mass w with its center (of mass) at r_x, r_y, r_z and its long axis in direction λ, μ, ν, the inertia tensor I_{wire} is

$$I_{wire} = W \begin{bmatrix} \tfrac{1}{3} d^2 (\mu^2 + \nu^2) + (r_y^2 + r_z^2) & -\tfrac{1}{3} d^2 (\lambda\mu) - (r_x r_y) & -\tfrac{1}{3} d^2 (\lambda\nu) - (r_x r_z) \\ -\tfrac{1}{3} d^2 (\lambda\mu) - (r_x r_y) & \tfrac{1}{3} d^2 (\lambda^2 + \nu^2) + (r_x^2 + r_z^2) & -\tfrac{1}{3} d^2 (\mu\nu) - (r_y r_z) \\ -\tfrac{1}{3} d^2 (\lambda\nu) - (r_x r_z) & -\tfrac{1}{3} d^2 (\mu\nu) - (r_y r_z) & \tfrac{1}{3} d^2 (\lambda^2 + \mu^2) + (r_x^2 + r_y^2) \end{bmatrix}$$

The sum of the tensors for the wires in the tree is the inertia tensor of the tree, whose principal planes and axes, with the dispersions about them, may be found by the methods mentioned in the last section. The second terms in I_{wire} are seen to be just an I_x, and represent inertia of the wire considered as a mass point. If the wires are mostly short compared to their distance from the origin, the resulting tensor will be closely approximated by that obtained by using the second terms alone. That is, each wire is approximated as a point mass located at the wire's C. of M.

At this point, we can go into some niceties of definition of "orientation" within the principal-axis framework and illustrate how different assumptions and definitions lead to different descriptions. We give an example of the principal-component calculation for two-dimensional wire trees. In two dimensions, hyperplanes and lines are the same thing; here only the inertia calculations are performed. Figure 1 shows the trees and, for each, four different sets of principal axes, illustrating that differences may arise from choices of approximation or origin of coordinates.

In two dimensions, the axes computed about a point away from the C. of M. either for wires or their approximating points will always be similar (axes A1 and A2, B1 and B2) since the best-fit line in either case passes through the C. of M. of the system. The similarity would not necessarily be so close in more dimensions.

On the other hand, the interpretation of moments around the center of mass should be done with care. Axes A3 arise from the approximation of branches by points, and indicate that the points are oriented in a single straight vertical line, i.e., there is a 0-error vertical line through the approximated branches, which is true. However, calculation of the moments around the C. of M. for wires, given in A4, indicates that there is not preferred orientation for a best-fit line; all moments through the C. of M. of the tree are equal. It is shaped "like a circle," not a line at all. Worse yet, neither of these opposite descriptions may be the one desired. It is easy to imagine that since the branches "point off to the right" from the branch point (which may be a scientifically interesting point, such as the soma of a neuron), the description should reflect this fact with a horizontal best-fit line, as provided by A1 and A2 in the first place.

The tree B serves again to show the differences induced by the point approximation (B3) and the wire moments (B4) about the C. of M. The approximation again claims both a better fit and a different direction than does the exact calculation.

It should be mentioned that with real automatically tracked neuron data the point approximation to wires seems very reasonable, and the choice of soma vs. C. of M. origin does not seem to make much difference (Figs. 2 and 3, Tables I and II).

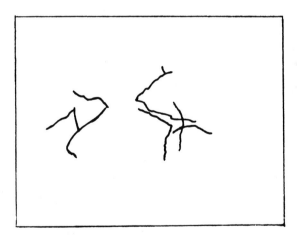

Fig. 2. Drawing from display of wire tree resulting from an automatic dendrite-tracking program. The z axis is out of the page. Moment calculations are done only for C. of M. of branches, and moments are relative (see Table I). The axis of minimum inertia is nearly parallel to the x axis, and from the moments it is seen that the neuron is relatively elongated in this direction. The elongation is less pronounced if axes are taken through the soma.

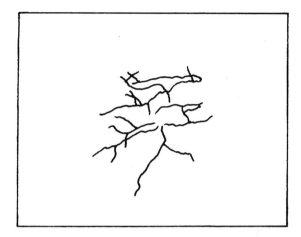

Fig. 3. Drawing from display of wire tree resulting from an automatic dendrite-tracking program, as in Fig. 2 (see Table II). The neuron is extended slightly in the 1 o'clock–7 o'clock direction, as seen by the direction of the axis of smallest inertial moment and the relative magnitudes of other axes. The elongation again appears greater if the C. of M. is taken as the origin rather than the soma.

Table I. Moment Calculations for Wire Tree in Fig. 2 (Mass = 464.78)[a]

Axis	Is	Ps	Axis direction cosines
1	1.00	1.79	(−0.965, 0.043, 0.255)
2	2.39	0.40	(0.234, 0.559, 0.795)
3	2.19	0.60	(0.108, −0.828, 0.550)

	Icm	Pcm	Axis direction cosines
1	1.00	2.11	(0.951, 0.053, −0.303)
2	2.58	0.53	(0.307, −0.234, 0.992)
3	2.64	0.47	(0.022, 0.970, 0.239)

[a]Is, Icm, moments about axis through soma and C. of M.; Ps, Pcm, moments about normal plane through soma and C. of M.

Table II. *Moment Calculations for Wire Tree in Fig. 3 (Mass = 694.77)[a]*

Axis	Is	Ps	Axis direction cosines
1	1.00	0.88	(−0.445, −0.878, 0.172)
2	1.55	0.33	(0.663, −0.194, 0.722)
3	1.21	0.67	(−0.600, 0.436, 0.669)
	Icm	Pcm	Axis direction cosines
1	1.00	1.085	(−0.500, −0.820, 0.275)
2	1.76	0.325	(−0.481, −0.000, −0.876)
3	1.41	0.675	(−0.719, 0.571, 0.394)

[a]See footnote to Table I for abbreviations.

3. Other Definitions of Orientation

Because of point weighting, the principal-components method gives no information as to the spatial extent of the structure it describes. Even if all points have equal weight, the dispersion numbers give a distorted (by the squared-distance dispersion measure) picture of the spatial extent of the structure. In order to obtain some idea of the actual spatial extent of the neuron, the following easy method, building on the principal-axis determination, is being implemented.

A right rectangular prism is constructed with faces parallel to the principal axes: thus the orientation of all six face planes is fixed. The exact location of each face plane is determined by choosing that location which puts $N\%$ of the structure's points on the "inside" side of the face plane ($N = 100$ for the maximum extent the neuron achieves). The whole construction takes only some distance calculations from points to the three "principal" planes (accomplished by dot products) and three sorts of the resulting signed distances.

The descriptions of orientation mentioned so far are very terse characterizations of global properties of the dendritic field. Another useful and complementary characterization of orientation is a statistical one, namely the orientation properties of the ensemble of individual wire segments in the wire tree. A system exists (Brown, 1976) which takes as input the wire tree data and which constructs and displays visualizations of the orientational properties of its wires. This description, based as it is on the elemental subparts of the wire tree, gives insight into the orientational "microstructure" of the dendrites rather than the orientational "macrostructure" characterized by the methods of this chapter.

ACKNOWLEDGMENTS

Prior work in finding two- and three-dimensional principal axes of point-swarm approximations to dendritic fields was done by C. F. Stephens and T. Walters, respectively, under P. D. Coleman. Thanks are due to N. Hogan for technical assistance. This research was sponsored by NSF/RANN Grant No. GI 34274X and Alfred P. Sloan Foundation Grant No. 74-12-5.

4. References

Brown, C. M., 1976, Representing the orientation of dendritic fields with geodesic tessellations, *TR13*, Computer Science Department, University of Rochester, Rochester, New York.

Businger, P. A., 1965, Algorithm 254; eigenvalues and eigenvectors of a real symmetric matrix by the QR method, *Commun. ACM* 8:218.

Garvey, C. F., Young, J. H., Jr., Coleman, P. D., and Simon, W., 1973, Automated three-dimensional dendrite tracking system, *Electroencephalogr. Clin. Neurophysiol.* 35:199.

Hubel, D. H., and Wiesel, T. N., 1962, Receptive fields, binocular interaction and functional architecture in two non-striate visual areas (18 and 19) of the cat, *J. Physiol. (London)* 160:106.

Pearson, K., 1901, On lines and planes of closest fit to systems of points in space, *Philosophical Magazine*, 6th ser., 2:559.

11

A Computerized Study
of Golgi-Impregnated Axons
in Rat Visual Cortex

A. Paldino and E. Harth

1. Introduction

In this chapter, we report preliminary results of a study on the structure of axons from pyramidal cells in the visual cortex (area 17) of albino rats. Measurements were taken with the video digitizer described in Chapter 3 of this volume. This instrument can be used to record spatial information on neuronal structure from a variety of tissue preparations displayed under a light microscope, but is most suited to the measurement of fiber trees as they appear in rapid Golgi or Golgi–Cox preparations.

Three-dimensional point information is stored on the disk of a PDP-10 computer. Different statistical parameters can then be extracted from this stored information, and orthogonal projections on planes of arbitrary orientation can be generated on a graphics terminal.

The study was undertaken to supplement the considerable body of information existing on the spatial distributions of apical and basal dendrites, particularly the quantitative investigations initiated by Sholl. A further rationale lies in a suggestion by Braitenberg (1974) that the clue to the origin of the linear receptive fields in the mammalian visual cortex may be found in axonal fine structure of cortical pyramids. One may make the following arguments: the transition from the roughly circular *spot detectors* encountered in the retina and

A. Paldino · Department of Neuroscience, Rose Fitzgerald Kennedy Center for Research in Mental Retardation and Human Development, Albert Einstein College of Medicine, Bronx, New York 10461. *E. Harth* · Physics Department, Syracuse University, Syracuse, New York 13210.

the lateral geniculate nuclei to the linear field structures observed in the cortex is usually attributed to selective connectivity between the latter two structures. A particular cortical neuron is assumed to receive afferents from geniculate spot detectors whose fields lie on a straight line. The evident cylindrical symmetry of both basal and apical dendrites would seem to place the burden of achieving the desired result on the spatial arrangement of afferent fibers or intermediary stellate neurons. In view of the many other requirements—retinotopic organization, ocular dominance columns, etc. — it is not clear what topology of fiber distribution in the plane of lamina IV would achieve these results. On the other hand, it is possible that the direct inputs to a particular pyramidal cell come from single geniculate spot detectors which leave their fiber endings arranged retinotopically in lamina IV. The observed linear receptive fields might then be due not to selective afferents but to *recurrent* interactions with neighboring pyramidal cells, producing cooperative effects among these cells. In this picture, the distribution of axon collaterals, especially anisotropies in azimuth angles, could play an important role in the shaping of cortical receptive fields.

2. Preliminary Considerations

We have utilized the rapid Golgi technique (including perfusion of the animal and embedding in celloidin) since this particular stain impregnates the entire axonal network of a neuron. The results to follow are from two albino rat brains, designated as sets A and B. Specimen A was 50 days old; the exact age of B was uncertain but known to be between 35 and 60 days. Both were immersed (after perfusion) in the rapid Golgi fixative for 3 days and in 0.75% silver nitrate for 2 days, embedded in celloidin, microtomed, and mounted on microslides with coverglasses. The resulting stain yielded a patchwork of impregnated neurons with their axonal trees. Slide 17 from set A and slide 3 from set B were chosen. By comparing their general cross-sectional features with drawings from Koenig and Klippel (1963), it was determined that these slides contained a large portion of the visual area (area 17).

The analysis of the data is preceded by the determination of a coordinate system to which all these data are common. A right-handed Cartesian system is used where the X coordinate indicates the focal *depth* in the tissue, the Z coordinate is in the direction perpendicular to the pial surface, and the Y coordinate represents an axis parallel to the pial surface. Figure 1 shows the orientation of this set of axes.

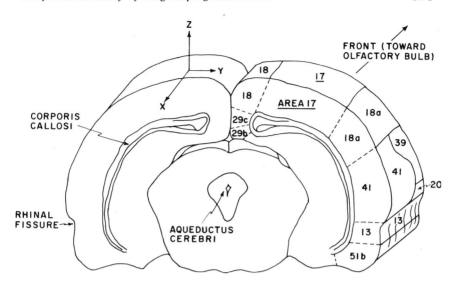

Fig. 1. Orientation of Cartesian coordinate system utilized in this study and location of area 17.

3. Structural Analysis of Axonal Networks

The axons analyzed are from 22 neurons in set A and 17 neurons in set B. Data collected from set A were obtained at 250x magnification, while the data from set B were obtained at 0.1 oil immersion (1000x magnification).

The distribution of the cell location at various depths below the pial surface is given in Figs. 2 and 3. All of these fibers studied belong to cells located in either layer III or layer IV with the exception of one deep pyramidal cell of layer V from set B. It should be pointed out that the cortical thickness of the two sets differs. In set A the cortex was estimated to be about 1000 μm thick, while the cortical thickness in set B was measured to be 1400 μm.

One of the most obvious features of interest in the axonal network is the angular distribution of its collaterals. The polar and azimuth angles were calculated for the initial segment of all collaterals. Collectively there are 153 collaterals from the 22 axons of set A, and 162 collaterals from the 17 axons of set B, indicating an average of 8.0 axon collaterals per cell. Figures 4, 5, and 6 show the azimuth angle distributions of axon collaterals, Fig. 7 gives the polar angle distribution, and Fig. 8 represents the cosine plot of the polar angle distribution.

The shape of the azimuth angle distribution for set A suggests maxima near 90° and 270°. There appear to be no pronounced maxima for set B, only a

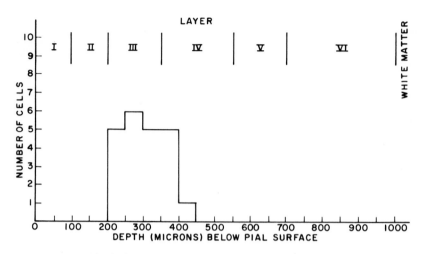

Fig. 2. Set A: Cell location vs. depth below pial surface.

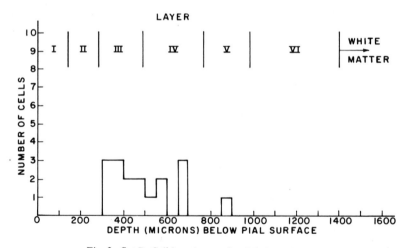

Fig. 3. Set B: Cell location vs. depth below pial surface.

weak minimum near 180°. Figure 6, which combines the data of the two sets, indicates a mild anisotropy for the azimuth angles of pyramidal cell axon collaterals favoring the 90° and 270° directions. Better statistics are required on this important point; in particular, one would have to examine carefully whether the apparent favoring of the sagittal plane is not due to our sectioning along that same plane.

Consider the polar angle distribution of these axon collaterals in Fig. 7. Here are represented the polar angles of the combined sets showing this distribution for 315 axon collaterals. Unmistakably there is a very strong maximum near 90° This is in part due to the larger solid angle per polar angle interval near 90°. Figure 8 shows the cosine plot for this distribution, which eliminates the geometric effect. It is seen that the maximum persists at an angle

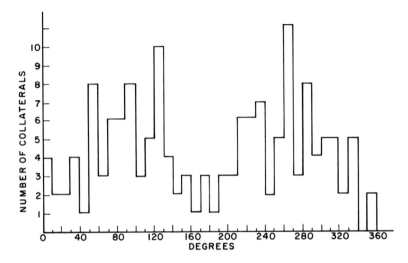

Fig. 4. Set A: Azimuth angle of collateral segment (total 153).

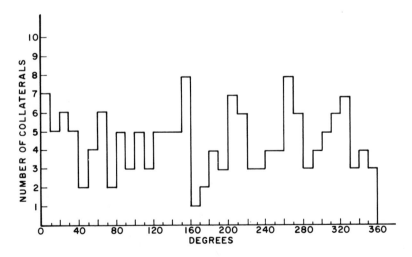

Fig. 5. Set B: Azimuth angle of collateral segment (total 162).

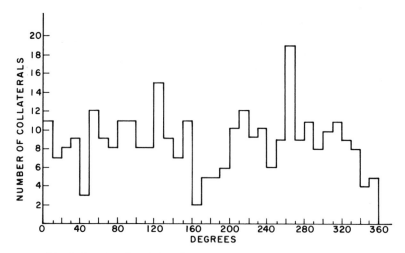

Fig. 6. Sets A and B: Azimuth angle of collateral segment (total 315).

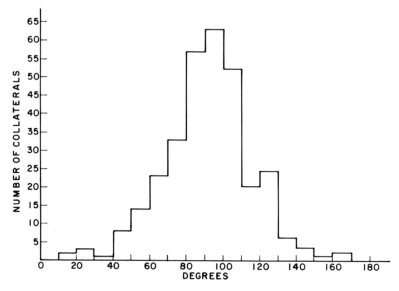

Fig. 7. Sets A and B: Polar angle of collateral segment (total 315).

slightly larger than 90°, indicating that these collaterals initially attempt to grow either parallel to the pial surface or slightly tilted toward deeper layers.

The terminal points of these axon collaterals are significant since they are probably sites of synapses with fibers from other cells. A meaningful azimuthal distribution of these terminals would have required us to follow each exiting fiber into neighboring sections until a terminal was found. This was not done in the present experiment, although we have developed a method for finding fiber continuations (Chapter 3). The graph of azimuth angles obtained from single sections in which we have counted exiting points *and* true fiber terminals is shown in Fig. 9 combining the data from both sets of neurons. The very pronounced maxima in the plane of the section (near 90° and 270°) are clearly

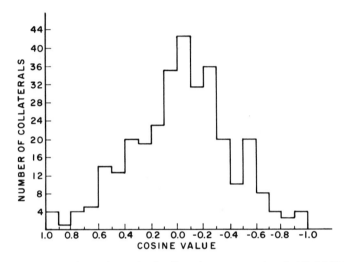

Fig. 8. Sets A and B: Polar angle of collateral segment, cosine plot (total 315).

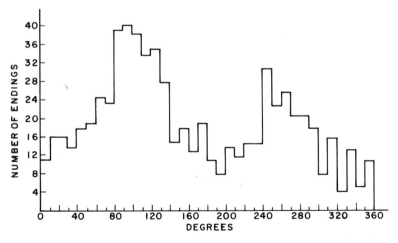

Fig. 9. Sets A and B: Azimuth angle of endings with respect to their cell location (total 688).

indicative of the fiber endings missed because of the finite thickness of the sections.

Since our sample includes cells from different regions of the striate cortex, any preferential orientation of individual axonal trees related to receptive field axes would be expected to be obscured. From this point of view, it appears more meaningful to examine the individual axonal branchings. Figures 10–13 show polar graphs of the azimuth angles of axonal end points. Each figure represents a single axonal tree. Several types of distribution were observed, suggesting a division into axonal classes. In Fig. 10 is shown an example of an axon in which all branches fall into a cone of less than 50°. Several cases were observed in which all branches terminated within two cones approximately 180° apart (Fig. 11), while others showed a more isotropic distribution (Fig. 13).

A critical feature in the analysis of end-point data is their position with respect to the pial surface. In this analysis, however, only points which terminate within the volume of tissue are considered; that is exiting points are not included. A total of 275 points are analyzed from set A (Fig. 14) and 235 points

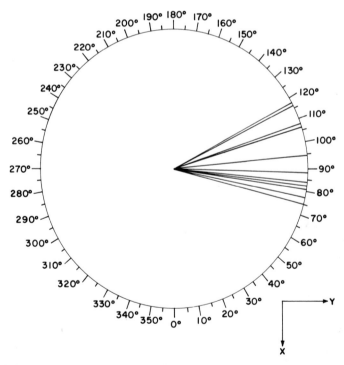

Fig. 10. Polar graph of axonal end points from fiber 11, set A. Example of divergence in one direction.

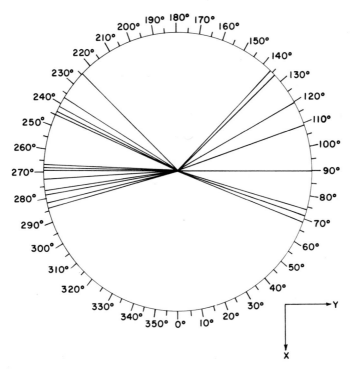

Fig. 11. Polar graph of axonal end points from fiber 17, set A. Example of divergence in two directions.

from set B (Fig. 15). Superimposed on each of these figures are the locations of the cell bodies from which these points arise. Note that the distribution of collateral end points of set B has a broad peak around 700 μm, while that of set A has two very distinct maxima, one at approximately 350 μm (lamina III–IV boundary) and a lesser but quite prominent one at approximately 700 μm (lamina V–VI boundary). The cell locations of set B are in different laminae (III, IV, and V), while those of set A are clustered in lamina III and (upper) lamina IV. Therefore, the broad peak of Fig. 15 is significant but not nearly as striking as peaks depicted in Fig. 14. These two maxima indicate that pyramidal cells located in lamina III and (upper) lamina IV have axon collateral terminals either in (lower) lamina III or in (lower) lamina V and (upper) lamina VI. The first maximum exists at and somewhat below the depth of the cell locations. This suggests that these pyramidals have a strong tendency to send their axons to cells at or below their own level: small pyramids, basket cells, and the "double dendritic bouquet" cells. The second maximum occurs approximately 350–400 μm deeper in the cortex. These latter terminals may contribute to the

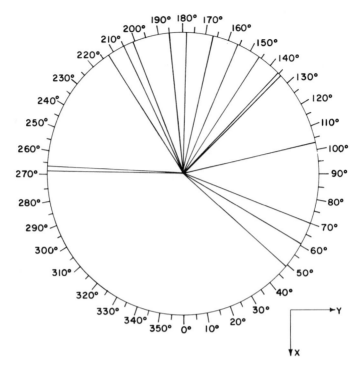

Fig. 12. Polar graph of axonal end points from fiber 12, set B. Example of void region.

stria of Baillarger, a tangential fiber plexus bordering (lower) lamina V and (upper) lamina VI, arising probably from horizontal collaterals of the deep pyramids and from axons or axon collaterals of the large layer IV stellates.

In Fig. 16 we have combined all data and sorted the end points according to the layer in which they are located. A single strong peak is seen in layer IV. Since this layer also represents the main input to the visual cortex from the specific sensory afferents from the lateral geniculate body, it appears that the sensory information which has reached these pyramidal neurons is fed back to layer IV and mixed with the direct visual inputs.

Another interesting feature is the location of these fiber terminals with respect to the cell body from which they arise. Let Z_T be the depth of the terminal points and Z_{CB} be the location of the cell body. We now consider a distribution of the number of endings as a function of the distance $Z_{CB} - Z_T$. Figures 17 and 18 depict this analysis for sets A and B, respectively. Note that the vast majority of these end points lie within 200 μm below the cell body and very few terminate above it. However, both sets of data indicate a subtle but discernible maximum at a lower level. For set A the minor peak is at approximately 450 μm, and for set B it is around 600 μm below the cell body, distances which are in the same ratio as the gray matter thicknesses (1000 and 1400 μm) of the two sets.

Of obvious interest is the lateral distribution of these end points. For this we consider the distance R in the *Y-Z* plane of all points ending within the tissue from their respective cell-body location, irrespective of the Z dimension. The number of endings decreases roughly exponentially as one moves laterally away from the cell body. The combined data (Fig. 20) show that the exponential distribution has a space constant of roughly 100 μm, indicating that lateral communication between cells is mostly short range. The average radius of all end points is 64 μm. These results agree with Chiang (1973), whose measurements indicate that the average axonal radius of pyramidal cells located in layers II–VI is less than 100 μm.

Finally, mention should be made of the integrated fiber lengths. Some fibers bifurcate very little, while others have very profuse branching. Total fiber lengths of all the 35 fibers (22 from set A and 13 from set B) range from a low of 413 μm to a high of 2876 μm. The average axonal length of the 35 fibers is

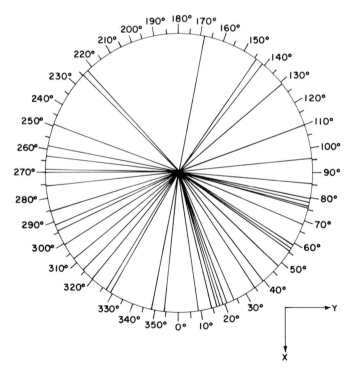

Fig. 13. Polar graph of axonal end points from fiber 6, set B. Example of anisotropy.

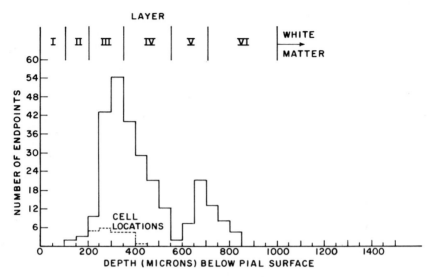

Fig. 14. Set A: End points vs. depth below pial surface (total 275).

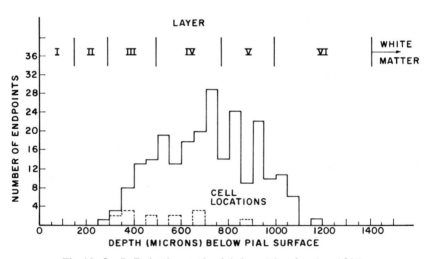

Fig. 15. Set B: End points vs. depth below pial surface (total 235).

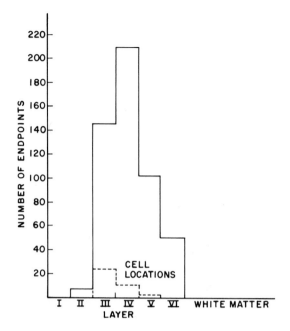

Fig. 16. Sets A and B: End points vs. layer location (total 510).

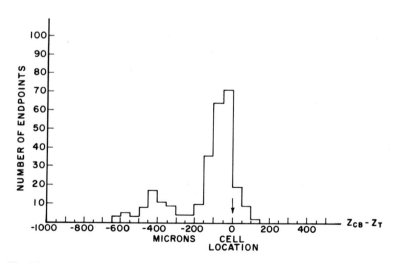

Fig. 17. Set A: Distance of end points from cell location in Z dimension (total 275).

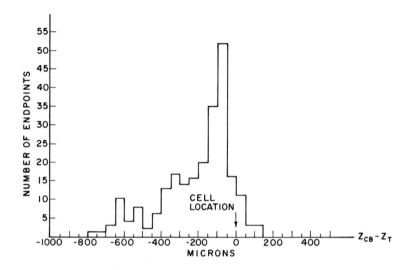

Fig. 18. Set B: Distance of end points from cell location in Z dimension (total 235).

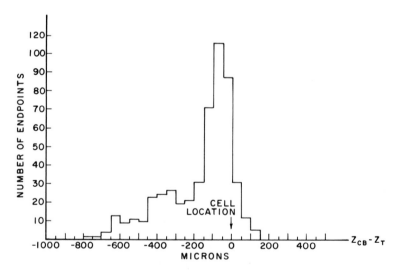

Fig. 19. Sets A and B: Distance of end points from cell location in Z dimension (total 510).

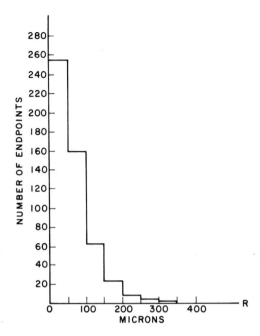

Fig. 20. Sets A and B: End points vs. distance (R) from cell location in X=Y plane (total 510).

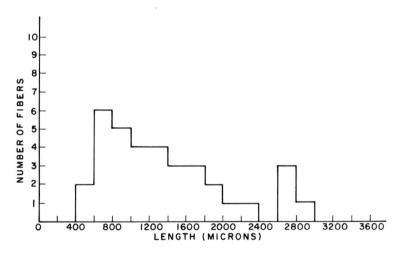

Fig. 21. Sets A and B: Integrated fiber lengths, (axon only) (total 35, average length 1376 μm).

PIAL SURFACE

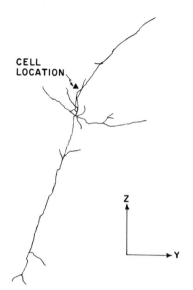

Fig. 22. Set A, fiber 1: Computer plot of visual display.

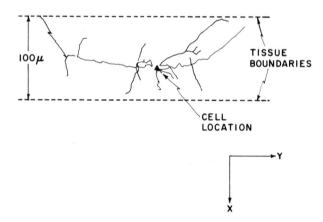

Fig. 23. Set A, fiber 1: Computer plot of visual display.

1376 μm. The distribution of the axonal lengths is shown in Fig. 21. It must be pointed out that these lengths are lower limits since fiber segments appearing in adjacent sections are not included.

A computer program reconstructs the three-dimensional data which are on disk and displays the fiber image on the PDP-10/VB10C graphics terminal of the Syracuse University Computing Center. On the terminal, the operator can

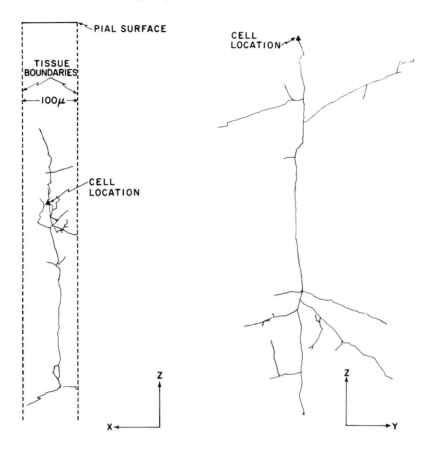

Fig. 24. Set A, fiber 1: Computer plot of visual display.

Fig. 25. Set A, fiber 17: Computer plot of visual display.

translate and rotate the image with respect to any of the three axes. The size of the image can be adjusted by activating, via a light pen, a scale bar superimposed on the graphics screen. The program also can plot, on the CALCOM (IBM 370/155 plotter), the image currently being displayed. Figure 22 is a plot of fiber 1 data from set A in the Z-Y plane. The horizontal line at the top of the figure indicates the pial surface. Figure 23 shows this same fiber rotated 90° about the Y axis so as to present the X-Y plane. In this view, the observer is looking "down" the main axonal shaft from the pial surface toward the white matter. The main shaft, however, diverges from the Z axis. Figure 24 shows this fiber displayed in the X-Z plane. Figures 25–27 show the reconstructed data of fiber 17 from set B.

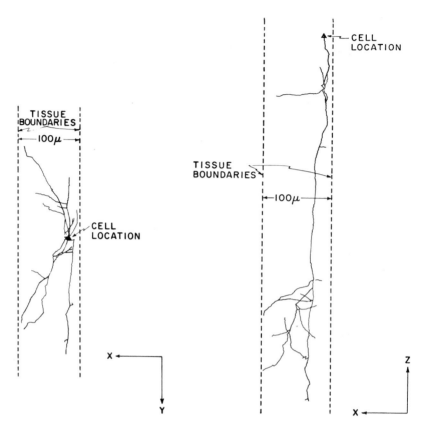

Fig. 26. Set A, fiber 17: Computer plot   Fig. 27. Set A, fiber 17: Computer plot
of visual display.   of visual display.

4. Conclusion

We have presented preliminary results of an ongoing study. Among the results that deserve mentioning is the finding that axon terminals for individual cells rarely show a uniform distribution in azimuth angle but as a rule have strong asymmetries and anisotropies. This finding lends some support to the supposition that cortical interconnectivity rather than afferent selectivity may account for the emergence of direction-sensitive cortical fields.

The radial separation of axon terminals from the cell body is found to approximate an exponential decay with a space constant of about 100 μm.

Visual displays aid the investigator in the determination of complex structures; for example, quick inspection of the axonal network at the appropriate orientation enables one to determine any asymmetries of end points, integrated fiber distances between any two fiber points, and symmetries or anisotropies of the axon collaterals. It is expected that this technique will become very useful as refinements are added.

ACKNOWLEDGMENTS

The authors wish to acknowledge the assistance of Mr. D. Carr for writing the computer program for the graphic displays and of Ms. B. Howden for preparing the illustrations. This research was supported in part by grant NS 10917 from The National Institutes of Health.

5. References

Braitenberg, V., 1974, Thoughts on the cerebral cortex, *J. Theor. Biol.* **46**:421–447.
Chiang, B., 1973, The organization of the visual cortex, doctoral dissertation, Syracuse University.
Hubel, D. H., and Wiesel, T. N., 1963, Shape and arrangement of columns in cat's striate cortex, *J. Physiol. (London)* **165**:559–570.
Hubel, D. H., and Wiesel, T. N., 1968, Receptive fields and functional architecture of monkey striate cortex, *J. Physiol. (London)* **195**:215–243.
Koenig, J. G. R.,and Klippel, R. A., 1963, *The Rat Brain: A Stereotaxic Atlas of the Forebrain and Lower Parts of the Brain Stem*, Williams and Wilkins, Baltimore.

Index